PEDIATRICS - LABORATORY AND CLINICAL RESEARCH

PEDIATRIC CANCER

PEDIATRICS - LABORATORY AND CLINICAL RESEARCH

Additional books in this series can be found on Nova's website under the Series tab.

Additional E-books in this series can be found on Nova's website under the E-book tab.

CANCER ETIOLOGY, DIAGNOSIS AND TREATMENTS

Additional books in this series can be found on Nova's website under the Series tab.

Additional E-books in this series can be found on Nova's website under the E-book tab.

PEDIATRICS - LABORATORY AND CLINICAL RESEARCH

PEDIATRIC CANCER

WILLIAM LI
EDITOR

Nova Science Publishers, Inc.
New York

For permission to use material from this book please contact us:
Telephone 631-231-7269; Fax 631-231-8175
Web Site: http://www.novapublishers.com

Additional color graphics may be available in the e-book version of this book.

LIBRARY OF CONGRESS CATALOGING-IN-PUBLICATION DATA

Pediatric cancer / editor, William Li.
p. cm.
Includes bibliographical references and index.
ISBN 978-1-61942-112-7 (hardcover)
1. Cancer in children. I. Li, William.
RC281.C4P363 2011
618.92'994--dc23

2011043200

Published by Nova Science Publishers, Inc. ✝ New York

CONTENTS

Preface **vii**

Acknowledgements **xvii**

Chapter 1 The Overview of Pediatric Cancer in Hong Kong **1**
Godfrey C. F. Chan

Chapter 2 The Impact of Cancer on the Psychosocial Well-Being and Quality of Life of Hong Kong Chinese Children **15**
William H. C. Li

Chapter 3 Effectiveness of Therapeutic Play Intervention in Promoting the Psychosocial Well-Being of Children Hospitalized with Cancer **31**
William H. C. Li

Chapter 4 Understanding how Children Coped with Cancer: An Essential Prerequisite for Designing Appropriate Psycho-Educational Interventions **55**
William H. C. Li

Chapter 5 The Psychosocial Well-Being and Quality of Life of Childhood Cancer Survivors: An Exploratory Study **75**
William H. C. Li

Chapter 6	Developing and Evaluating an Empowerment Programme in Promoting the Psychosocial Well-Being and Quality of Life of Childhood Cancer Survivors: A Pilot Study *William H. C. Li*	**97**
Chapter 7	Psychosocial Support for Parents of Children with Cancer *Sau-ying Chiu and Eva K. Y. Ho*	**119**
Chapter 8	Continuous Renal Replacement Therapy in Children Post-Hematopoietic Stem Cell Transplantation *Lama Elbahlawan and R. Ray Morrison*	**133**
Index		**149**

PREFACE

The diagnosis and treatment of cancer can be a stressful and threatening experience, particularly for children. This book will shed light on the impact of cancer and its treatments on the physical, emotional, and psychosocial well-being of both children hospitalized with cancer and childhood cancer survivors. Additionally, this book will explore the coping strategies used by children with cancer and their parents. This book reports some empirical studies on evaluating the effectiveness of various psychological interventions in promoting the psychosocial well-being and quality of life of children with cancer. It is anticipated that this book can provide readers a more thorough understanding about the impact of cancer on children's physical and psychological well-being.

Chapter 1 - Although cancer is relatively rare in children, it seriously affects the physical well-being of children. Cancer is the 2nd most common cause of death in children and may lead to long term disability in Hong Kong. There are quite a number of misconceptions on childhood cancer. Some people may not be able to distinguish the fundamental differences between the adult cancer and childhood cancer. In fact, childhood cancers seldom develop from epithelial of glandular tissues, which are contrary to the adult cancers. Therefore, topographic classification is not a meaningful approach in childhood cancer. Additionally, although most childhood cancers have genetic aberrations found in the tumor tissue, it is due to mutation occurs during the child's development rather than passing of genetic abnormalities from parents to the child. Furthermore, more should be done to investigate the variation of distribution of types of malignancy in different ethnic groups. With the advancement in treatment modalities, around 70% of all children with cancers can be cured in most developed countries. The new treatment modalities include intensity modulated radiation therapy (IMRT), image guided radiation therapy (IGRT or TOMO-RT) and minimal invasive approach with endoscopic method to perform biopsy or tumor excision, which can improve the survival rate of children. Another area of concern in the field of childhood cancers is pediatric palliative care. Childhood hospice facility is a rarity in most countries including some developed and undeveloped countries. The end results are that unnecessary aggressive therapies are often applied up to the very last moment. In fact, pediatric palliative care is essential to relief the patients and their families from the unnecessary suffering and should be emphasized in future comprehensive pediatric care. In summary, a well designed treatment protocols and new treatment modalities drastically improved the outcome. With multidisciplinary approaches, respectable prognosis is expected. But a significant number of cancer survivors may have residual or late morbidity and requires long term follow-up monitoring. For a small proportion of children with incurable cancers, pediatric palliative care should be provided to make the patients and their families sailing through the end of life journey with less suffering.

Chapter 2 - The diagnosis and treatment of cancer can be a stressful and threatening experience, particularly for children. Although survival rates are higher than ever as a result of new technology and breakthroughs in cancer treatment, the course of treatment for cancer is still a very stressful experience in the life of a child. Unfortunately, most research in childhood cancer has traditionally concentrated on medical issues, and has disregarded the importance of the emotional and psychosocial well-being of children with cancer. Furthermore, most studies of childhood cancer conducted in Hong Kong have focused on examining the psychological well-being and quality of life of family members or caregivers. A review of the literature reveals that so far very few studies have attempted to investigate the experience of cancer from children's own perspectives in Hong Kong Chinese context. The aim of this chapter is to shed light on the psychosocial well-being and quality of life in Hong Kong Chinese children hospitalized with cancer based on the findings of two recent studies. Study One: The objective of Study One was to examine the impact of cancer on Hong Kong Chinese children's physical, emotional, and psychosocial well-being. A cross-sectional study was employed. Ninety-eight Hong Kong Chinese children aged 7 to 15 years, admitted for treatment of cancer in 2 paediatric oncology units of 2 different hospitals, were invited to participate in the study. Participants were asked to respond to the Chinese version of the State Anxiety Scale and the Center for Epidemiologic Studies Depression Scale for Children during hospitalization. Besides, a brief semi-structured interview was conducted with each participant before discharge home. Study Two: The objective of study two was to explore the relationships among treatment-related symptoms, depressive symptoms and quality of life of Chinese children hospitalized with cancer. A cross-sectional study was employed. One hundred and thirty-five Hong Kong Chinese children aged 9 to 16 years, admitted for treatment of cancer in a paediatric oncology unit, were invited to participate in the study. Participants were asked to respond to the Chinese version of the Center for Epidemiologic Studies Depression Scale for Children (CES-DC) and the Chinese version of the Pediatric Quality of Life Inventory ™ (PedsQL™) Cancer Module. Additionally, each participant was asked to report the number and severity of the treatment-related symptoms that they experienced. The results of Study One showed that children reported considerably high state anxiety scores on admission for treatment of cancer. Besides, semi-structured interviews revealed that nearly all children expressed different degrees of sadness and worry. Additionally, findings from this study indicated that more than half of the participants were potentially at risk for depression, or at least presented some depressive symptoms during their stay in the hospital. The results of Study Two indicated that there were high correlations between treatment-related symptoms and quality of life, treatment-related symptoms and depressive symptoms, and depressive symptoms and quality of life, with children reporting greater symptom severity experiencing higher levels of depression and a lower level of quality of life. These two studies have addressed a gap in the literature by investigating the experience of cancer, in particular the quality of life from children's own perspectives in Hong Kong Chinese context. The results reveal that cancer has tremendous impact on children's physical, emotional, psychosocial well-being and quality of life. There is an imperative need for nurses to evaluate appropriate nursing interventions that can help children ease the burden of cancer treatment, enhance their quality of life and provide support for them to fight cancer at every step of their long and difficult journey.

Chapter 3 - Childhood cancer and its treatment have been described as an extremely stressful and threatening experience, which can be emotionally devastating for children. Although survival rates for childhood cancer are higher than ever before, the course of treatment for cancer, such as chemotherapy, surgery or radiotherapy, is still a very stressful experience in the life of a child. Children with cancer may not only be at risk from adverse medical effects; their psycho-social well being may also be severely affected as a result of the cancer and its therapy. The aims of this study were to examine the effectiveness of therapeutic play using virtual reality computer games, in minimizing anxiety and reducing depressive symptoms in Hong Kong Chinese children hospitalized with cancer. Specifically whether a virtual reality computer game is feasible to be implemented in clinical settings and acceptable to health care providers, children hospitalized with cancer and their parents were the focus. A non-equivalent control group pretest-posttest, between-subject design was employed. Hong Kong Chinese Children (8-16 years of age), admitted to two paediatric oncology units of two different regional acute public hospitals in Hong Kong during a 16-month period, were invited to participate in the study. Of the 133 children, 72 formed the control group receiving routine information preparation and 61 in the experimental group receiving therapeutic play using virtual reality computer games. The results showed that children in the experimental group reported statistically significant fewer depressive symptoms than children in the control group on day 7. The results, however, although children in the experimental group had lower mean state anxiety scores than children in the control group on day 7, the differences were not statistically significant. The study provides empirical evidence to support the effectiveness, feasibility and acceptability of using virtual reality computer games in the psychological preparation of children hospitalized with cancer, thus charting a path towards promoting holistic and quality care. It is anticipated that the findings of this empirical study will promote awareness in nurses and parents that play is a very important part of children's life, and that they need play even when they are ill. Additionally, the findings will contribute to promoting nurses' accountability and responsibility for patient care through evidence-based practice.

Chapter 4 - Notwithstanding the increasing survival rates for childhood cancers, the course of treatment for cancer, such as chemotherapy, surgery or radiotherapy, is still a very stressful experience in the life of a child and may lead to long term physical, emotional and psychosocial damage for children. There is some evidence that both chemotherapy and radiotherapy may have adverse effects upon normal body tissue that may manifest themselves months or even years after completion of the therapy. However, children with cancer may not only be at risk from adverse medical effects, their psycho-social well being, self-esteem and quality of life may also be severely affected as a result of their cancer and its therapy. There is an imperative need for nurses to develop and evaluate interventions that can help to ease the burden of cancer treatment for children. First, however, knowing how children coped with the diagnosis and treatment of cancer is a crucial step toward designing appropriate psycho-educational interventions. A cross-sectional study was employed. Eighty-eight Hong Kong Chinese children aged 9 to 16 years, admitted for treatment of cancer in a paediatric oncology unit of an acute public hospital, were invited to participate in the study. To understand how children coped with their illness and responded to the diagnosis and treatment of cancer, they were asked to respond to the Coping Behaviour Checklist for Chinese Children on day 7 after admission or before discharge. The results of this study revealed that Hong Kong Chinese children and their Western counterparts adopted different strategies for coping with cancer. The findings indicated that self-control (emotion-focused) was the most commonly reported coping strategy used by Hong Kong Chinese children. The results of this study is incongruent with previous studies on Western children in which it was found that seeking social support (problem-focused) was the most commonly reported coping strategy. On the other hand, this study revealed that children used different coping strategies at different developmental stages, with younger children (aged 9-12) used less problem-focused and more emotion-focused coping strategies than older children (aged 13-16). An understanding of the coping behaviour of children is an essential prerequisite for the design of an appropriate psycho-educational intervention to reduce the children's emotional distress and bolster their coping mechanisms. This study has addressed a gap in the literature by examining how Hong Kong Chinese children coped with and responded to the diagnosis and treatment of cancer. It is anticipated that the information derived from this study can make a contribution to the advancement of nursing knowledge. Most importantly, the findings from this study can help nurses to shape and design appropriate psychological interventions that can help to reduce the burden of the cancer treatment and promote normal growth and development for children with cancer.

Chapter 5 - Recent advances in cancer screening and medical treatment for childhood cancer have dramatically improved survival rates. Yet, despite the improved prognosis, cancer survivors have to pay a high price in side effects, such as second malignancies, growth and endocrine dysfunction, and serious organ toxicities. Most of these health problems are considered late-emerging side effects of the chemotherapy and radiation treatments, which may manifest months or even years after the completion of treatment, severely affecting children's psychosocial well-being and quality of life. Whilst much of the effort has been paid to the physiological care of childhood cancer survivors, insufficient attention has focused on the impact of cancer and its treatment on the psychosocial well-being of childhood cancer survivors in Hong Kong. The aim of this study was to examine the impact of cancer on the psychosocial well-being and quality of life of Hong Kong Chinese childhood cancer survivors, an area of research that has been underrepresented in the literature. To examine the impact of cancer on children, a cross-section study was employed. A total of 137 childhood cancer survivors, aged 9 to 16 years old, who had their medical follow-up at the out-patient clinic were invited to participate in the study. Participants were asked to respond to the Chinese version of the Centre for Epidemiologic Studies Depression Scale for Children, Rosenberg's Self-Esteem Scale and Pediatric Quality of Life Inventory. Additionally, a one-to-one qualitative interview was conducted with 10 participants randomly selected from the group. The results of the study indicated that more than half of the participants were potentially at risk for depression, or at least presented some depressive symptoms. There were high negative correlations between depressive symptoms and self-esteem scores, and depressive symptoms scores and level of quality of life. Furthermore, a medium positive correlation was found between self-esteem scores and level of quality of life. The findings indicated that greater depressive symptoms reported by childhood cancer survivors were associated with lower self-esteem and poorer quality of life. Additionally, the study revealed that depressive symptoms are a strong predictor of quality of life of childhood cancer survivors. The study reveals that cancer and its treatments have a tremendous impact on the psychosocial well-being and quality of life of survivors. It is essential for health care professionals to develop and evaluate appropriate interventions with the aims of promoting psychosocial well-being and enhancing the quality of life for these children. Most importantly, it is crucial to help them develop a positive view of the impact that the cancer experience has upon their life.

Chapter 6 - With advances in cancer screening and treatment, the survival rates for childhood cancer are higher than ever before. Yet, the course of treatment for cancer may lead to long term physical, emotional and psychosocial damage for children. Whilst much of the attention has focused on the physiological outcomes of cancer treatments in Hong Kong, the psychosocial well-being and quality of life of childhood cancer survivors have been disregarded or underestimated. Although various psychosocial interventions conducted in Western countries have shown beneficial effects on the psychosocial well-being of childhood cancer survivors, no similar intervention has been conducted in Hong Kong. Given to the different cultural background, it is uncertain whether the psychosocial interventions recommended by the Western literature can be appropriate for use in Hong Kong Chinese context. The aim of this chapter is to report a pilot study on developing and evaluating an empowerment programme for Hong Kong primary school students. A pilot study of a randomized controlled trial, two-group pre-test and repeated post-test, between-subjects design was employed in two primary schools. A convenience sampling of 120 primary school students was recruited of whom 56 were randomly assigned to the experimental group participating in the empowerment programme and 64 to the control group receiving continuous assessment of their psychosocial well-being and quality of life. All the participants were asked to response to the Center for Epidemiologic Studies Depression Scale for Children, Rosenberg's Self-Esteem Scale and Pediatric Quality of Life Inventory across the three time periods: at the time of recruitment (T1: pre-intervention), and at six months (T2) and 12 months (T3) after starting the intervention. The results of mixed between-within subjects ANOVA indicated that children in the experimental group reported statistically significant fewer depressive symptoms and higher self-esteem than children in the control group. The findings added further evidence that children who engaged in a healthy lifestyle, eating healthily and exercising regularly, reported fewer depressive symptoms and higher levels of self-esteem than those who did not engage in such a lifestyle. Furthermore, teaching children problem-solving and interpersonal skills, as well as how to cope with stress and adversity, it can enhance their psychosocial well-being and strengthen their resilience to psychological distress. Most importantly, this study has demonstrated the feasibility of implementing the empowerment programme in the Hong Kong Chinese context. The content, nature and duration of the empowerment programme were found to be acceptable by Hong Kong Chinese children and their parents. Therefore, it is anticipated that with some minor modifications, the empowerment programme can be used as an appropriate psychosocial interventions to promote psychosocial well-being and quality of life of Hong Kong Chinese childhood cancer survivors. In addition, health care professionals should set up a community supporting network for children with cancer and their family so that children can better combat with adverse psychosocial effects of cancer and its subsequent adverse treatment effects at every step of their long and difficult journey.

Chapter 7 - Cancer is a life-threatening disease. The physical and psychological well-being of children with cancer is detrimentally influenced by the disease. It is not only the children who suffer from the disease as cancer also exerts negative influences on the patients' families. A review of the literature reveals that the parents who have children with cancer carry heavy burdens of care and responsibility. However, there are only few studies that discuss the life experience of the parents who have children with cancer. In this chapter, we will explore different coping mechanisms, hospital and community resources that are being utilized by parents who have children with cancer in eastern countries, in particular, Hong Kong. Study: The objective of the study was to explore the life experience of parents who have chidren with cancer. For the purpose of this study, six mothers who are the primary caregivers were specifically selected from a paediatric oncology ward of a hospital. A semi-structured interview was conducted with each participant by a research nurse in the clinical area. The results of the study showed that parents adopted emotion focused coping strategies in dealing with challenges. They were influenced by the fatalism and concept of a sense of personal honour. In addition, they also adopted problem focused coping strategies in order to control the situation. Different interventions which include counseling services, patient education, parent support group, assisting them to mobilize social support and providing spiritual support should be implemented in the clinical setting. It is essential for nurses to understand the coping strategies being utilized by parents, so as to design and evaluate appropriate nursing interventions that can enhance parents' abilities to cope with the challenges.

Chapter 8 - Allogeneic hematopoietic stem cell transplantation (HSCT) is being utilized increasingly as a curative therapy for an array of disorders like hematologic malignancies, immunodeficiency, and inborn errors of metabolism. However, many complications that occur after transplant can have a significant negative impact on outcome and thus limit the benefit of this therapy. Acute renal failure (ARF) occurs commonly after HSCT and is associated with high risk of morbidity and mortality. Common factors associated with ARF early after HSCT include acute tubular necrosis, veno-occlusive disease, and septic shock. Conditioning regimens and total body irradiation as well as the use of nephrotoxic medications contribute to the occurrence of ARF 60 days following HSCT. Recently, continuous renal replacement therapy (CRRT) has emerged as the favored modality of renal replacement therapy in the care of critically ill children who are hemodynamically unstable. CRRT is increasingly used in the care of critically ill post-HSCT children to treat renal failure or to prevent fluid overload (FO) as FO seems to be associated with worse outcome in these patients. Studies have shown that the risk of mortality is higher when CRRT is initiated at FO>20% in critically ill children as well as post-HSCT children. In our experience, CRRT results in improved oxygenation in post-HSCT children with acute lung injury. Mean airway pressure at the end of CRRT seems to be an important prognostic factor for pediatric stem cell recipients who are mechanically ventilated because survivors have lower mean airway pressures at the end of CRRT compared to non-survivors. This high mean airway pressure at the end of CRRT is likely related to the intrinsic pulmonary process that lead to pulmonary failure rather than pulmonary edema secondary to FO. Although CRRT is associated with improved short-term outcome, long-term survival (>6 months following intensive care unit discharge) is very poor. Factors associated with lower long-term survival include higher C-reactive protein (CRP) and lower absolute neutrophil count (ANC). Prospective multi-institutional studies are needed to definitively establish prognostic factors associated with better survival. In addition, the best modality of CRRT for attenuating the inflammatory process should be investigated in this population. Protocols that delineate the appropriate time to initiate CRRT before 20% FO may also be valuable in improving outcome in this high-risk population.

ACKNOWLEDGEMENTS

The editor wishes to thank the NOVA Science Publishers, Inc. for allowing and supporting the publication of this book. Without the publishers' support, we cannot have adequate care, quality and design in the preparation of this book. The editor would also like to thank the authors of each chapter for their support and invaluable insights to different topics of interest and focus of this book – Pediatric Cancer. The research methods, findings and discussion provided by the authors would certainly make new and better understanding of pediatric cancer, particularly in Chinese populations.

I would like to express my utmost gratitude to Professor Godfrey Chi-Fung Chan, for his expertise, insightful suggestions, and constant inspiration throughout the preparation process of this book. Additionally, Professor Chan is kindly agreed to give his expert opinion on the topic of pediatric cancer by contributing a chapter for this book despite of his busy schedules in taking care of his pediatric cancer patients, administrative and research works. Professor Chan graduated from dentistry (1981) and medicine (1985) respectively in the Philippines and is currently both a registered dentist and medical doctor in Hong Kong. He joined the Department of Paediatrics & Adolescent Medicine (UPAM) of the University of Hong Kong (HKU) in 1989 and began his training in paediatric haematology / oncology in 1991. Then he pursued further training at the St. Jude Children's Research Hospital, USA as a fellow from 1993 to 1996. He then obtained Dip of Palliative Medicine (1997) from University of Wales and MSc from University of Birmingham (1999). He joined the Faculty of Medicine, University of Hong Kong as Clinical Associate Professor in 1999. He was appointed as the Assistant Dean (External Affair) of the LKS Faculty of Medicine in 2004 and Clinical Professor in 2009. He has published more than 190 full articles and obtained multiple prestigious International Awards (ANR, SIOP, ASPR, Endeavor Executive Award-Austrian Government) for his works on childhood neurogenic tumours and stem cells research.

I owe a great deal to the children and their parents who have shared their time, and their hearts for participating in the research reported in this book for what they have given can never be valued. Last but not least, the editor would like to express his thanks to his research assistant, Ms Ho Ka Yan, for her assistance in checking the format and references of all chapters in this book.

In: Pediatric Cancer
Editor: William Li
ISBN: 978-1-61942-112-7

Chapter 1

THE OVERVIEW OF PEDIATRIC CANCER IN HONG KONG

Godfrey C. F. Chan
Department of Paediatrics, Li Ka Shing Faculty of Medicine
The University of Hong Kong, Hong Kong S.A.R., China

ABSTRACT

Although cancer is relatively rare in children, it seriously affects the physical well-being of children. Cancer is the 2nd most common cause of death in children and may lead to long term disability in Hong Kong.

There are quite a number of misconceptions on childhood cancer. Some people may not be able to distinguish the fundamental differences between the adult cancer and childhood cancer. In fact, childhood cancers seldom develop from epithelial of glandular tissues, which are contrary to the adult cancers. Therefore, topographic classification is not a meaningful approach in childhood cancer. Additionally, although most childhood cancers have genetic aberrations found in the tumor tissue, it is due to mutation occurs during the child's development rather than passing of genetic abnormalities from parents to the child. Furthermore, more should be done to investigate the variation of distribution of types of malignancy in different ethnic groups.

With the advancement in treatment modalities, around 70% of all children with cancers can be cured in most developed countries. The new treatment modalities include intensity modulated radiation therapy (IMRT), image guided radiation therapy (IGRT or TOMO-RT) and minimal invasive approach with endoscopic method to perform biopsy or tumor excision, which can improve the survival rate of children.

Another area of concern in the field of childhood cancers is pediatric palliative care. Childhood hospice facility is a rarity in most countries including some developed and undeveloped countries. The end results are that unnecessary aggressive therapies are often applied up to the very last moment. In fact, pediatric palliative care is essential to relief the patients and their families from the unnecessary suffering and should be emphasized in future comprehensive pediatric care.

In summary, a well designed treatment protocols and new treatment modalities drastically improved the outcome. With multidisciplinary approaches, respectable prognosis is expected. But a significant number of cancer survivors may have residual or late morbidity and requires long term follow-up monitoring. For a small proportion of children with incurable cancers, pediatric palliative care should be provided to make the patients and their families sailing through the end of life journey with less suffering.

INTRODUCTION

Cancer is relatively rare in children. Its annual incidence is around 150 to 300/million children depending on the inclusion of children between 15 to 18 years or not [1, 2]. In Hong Kong, the children population (≤15 years) is around 1.1 million and therefore we have approximately 160 to 190 newly diagnosed cases of childhood cancers each year (Chan GCF, HKPHOSG Annual Workshop 2011). Comparing to adult cancers with an annual incidence of around 25,000 in Hong Kong based on the Hong Kong Cancer Registry Report, the number of childhood cancer is apparently very small (<1% of adult cancers) (Figure 1). However, cancer is the 2nd most common cause of death in children, just next to accident [3, 4]. In addition, some forms childhood cancer, even if successfully treated, may lead to long term disability (i.e. brain tumors or bone tumors). Therefore, childhood cancer still accounts for a significant medical burden in any healthcare system.

There are also quite a number of misconceptions on childhood cancer. Many people try to extrapolate the concepts of adult cancer to childhood cancer but not aware of the fundamental differences between the two. More than 90% of adult cancers are derived from epithelial or glandular tissues, commonly known as carcinoma.

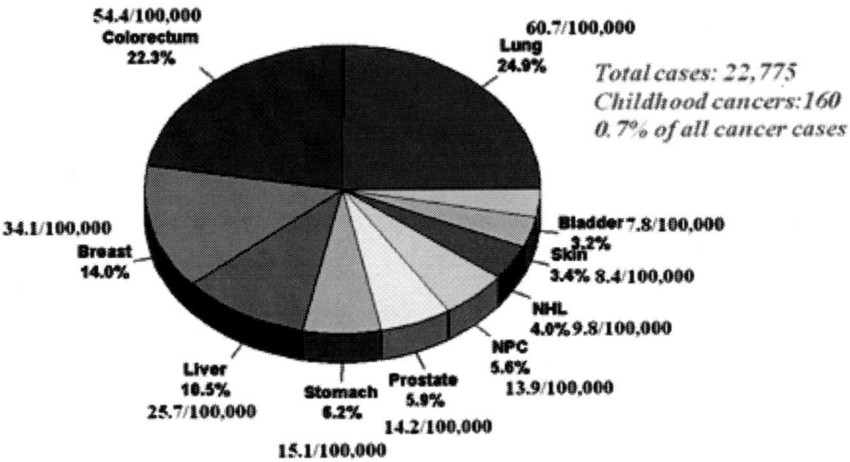

Figure 1. Most Common Cancers for All Ages in Both Sex (HK Cancer Registry 2005).

They are classified topographically by the location of the cancer such as head and neck, breast, nasopharynx, lung, liver, colon, etc. Many of them are developed from dysplastic tissues which evolved from either chronic inflammation or environment carcinogens. They often have a long latency period and screening may help to prevent them from progressing to advanced stage. Surgical resectability is a major outcome determinant for most of these cancers since their response to chemotherapy is generally not as good. In contrary, childhood cancers seldom develop from epithelial of glandular tissues. Lymphoid malignancy such as leukemia and lymphoma is the most common types of cancers in pediatric age group. The other cancers commonly found in children are solid tumors derived from either embryonal tissues such as blastoma (i.e. neuroblastoma, nephroblastoma, etc.) or from primitive mesenchymal tissues in the form of sarcoma (i.e. rhabdomyosarcoma, osteogenic sarcoma). The same type of tumor can be found in various parts of the body such as rhabdomyosarcoma can be found in the head and neck, extremities, pelvic cavity or the trunk region. Therefore, topographic classification is not a meaningful approach. Childhood cancers also has short latency period so screening will not be helpful. Many childhood cancers are aggressive in nature but paradoxically, they are more responsive to chemotherapy so in some situation, surgery may not be even needed (i.e. lymphoma). In general, around 70% of childhood cancers can be cured nowadays I developed countries (Table 1).

Table 1. Differences Between Childhood and Adult Cancers

Characteristics of Cancer	Adult	Children
Major Cancer Types	Carcinoma	Leukemia, Blastoma, Sarcoma
Common Sites	Superficial & Visible (i.e. breast, thyroid)	Deeply seated
Stage at Diagnosis	Can be early	Usually advanced
Screening	May help	Not effective
Response to treatment	Poor	Good
Overall outcome	20 to 30% Survive	70% Survive

Some frequently asked questions by the parents on childhood cancers are: 1) Are childhood cancers mostly inherited? 2) Is environmental toxins or infectious agents a major contributor of childhood cancer pathogenesis? 3) Will childhood cancer transmit to other siblings in the family? The current data suggests that while most childhood cancers have genetic aberrations found in the tumor tissue, that is due to mutation occurs during the child's development rather than passing of genetic abnormalities from parents to the child. Hereditary predisposition to cancer development only accounts for less than 10% of childhood cancer [5]. There are quite a number of studies suggest environmental carcinogens can lead to adult cancer development. But due to the relatively short incubation period, environmental factors do not play a major role in the pathogenesis of most childhood cancers[6]. Some specific viral agents such as Epstein Barr virus (EBV) surely can lead to lymphoid cells transformation and cancer development in childhood (i.e. endemic form of Burkitt lymphoma [7], mixed cellularity form of Hodgkin lymphoma [8]). Such situation is even more pronounced in children with underlying immunodeficiency [9, 10]. The other example is hepatitis associated hepatocellular carcinoma [11]. But after universal hepatitis vaccine has been given to all newborns in Hong Kong and Taiwan since 80's, a drastic decrease in the incidence of childhood hepatocellular carcinoma was noted. Aside from EBV and hepatitis B virus, there are some evidences to link viral infection to leukemia development.

Table 2. The Incidence of Childhood Cancer among Hong Kong Chincese Children

	(/million children ≤15 yrs)	
	HK	SEER (75-95)
• Acute leukaemia	42.1	45.6
• Brain tumors	31.2	36.2
• Non-Hodgkin lymphoma	9.8	14.5
• Extracranial germ cell tumor	7.9	5.4
• Neuroblastoma	5.3	9.1
• Rhabdomyosarcoma	5.0	4.6
• Osteosarcoma	4.8	4.8
• Ewing sarcoma / peripheral PNET	1.4/(2.8)	2.9/(N.A.)
• Hepatoblastoma	2.8	1.4
• Nephroblastoma (Wilm's tumor)	2.4	7.9

* http://seer.cancer.gov/publications/childhood/

For example, delayed exposure to some common viral pathogens may increase the chance of leukemia development in children [12]. In addition, seasonal variations of viral infections outbreak in a population seem to link with leukemic occurrence [13-15]. But it appears that viral infection per se may not be able explain the whole picture. It was found that some signature genetic abnormalities of leukemia can be found in more than 50% of children at birth even they develop leukemia in later childhood or adolescent period [16]. All of these data combined suggest that virus and intrinsic immunity plays a significant role in leukemic pathogenesis, especially for those patients already harbor the leukemic predisposed genes. With the exception of intrauterine transmission of leukemic clone in monozygotic twin, up to now, there is no evidence to suggest that childhood cancers can be transmitted either actively or passively from one child to the other like infectious disease does.

While the overall incidence of childhood cancers of different ethnic groups may be similar, the distribution of different types of malignancy varies significantly. For example, in central Africa, endemic form of Burkitt lymphoma is the most common form of childhood cancer [7] whereas in most of the other ethnic groups, acute lymphoblastic leukemia (ALL) accounts for >1/3 of childhood cancers. Ewing sarcoma of the bone is rare in Black population [17]. For Chinese and East Asian, much more germ cell tumors can be found when compare to the other ethnic groups (Table 2). But on the other hand, Chinese has much less Ewing sarcoma and Wilm tumor (nephroblastoma) than the Caucasian and Hispanic races. What may account for such variations remains to be unfolded. With the rapid progress in genetic methodology, the underlying mechanisms of such ethnic variation may soon be known.

The advancements in treatment modalities also change the prognosis of many childhood cancers in the past 2 decades. In general, around 70 to 80% of all children with cancers can be cured in most developed countries nowadays [18]. For the most common childhood cancer ALL, the long term survival can reach 80% mostly with chemotherapy alone [19-21]. By combining good treatment stratification based on risk factors and intensive intrathecal therapy, most ALL patients no longer require cranial irradiation [22]. The current success in ALL treatment is mainly due to the improvement in the usage of existing chemotherapeutic agents through sequential international collaborated clinical trials. This highlighted the importance of how we can move forward with well designed clinical trials. Using similar trial approach, significant progresses can also be found in Wilm tumor (i.e. NWS trials); rhabdomyosarcoma (i.e. IRS trials); lymphoma (i.e. LMB trials), etc. Currently, more than 90% of patient with Wilm's tumors [23]; more than 70% of patients with rhabdomyosarcoma [24-26] and more than 80% of patients with lymphoma [27, 28] can be cured. In addition to the proper use of chemotherapeutic agents, the improvement in surgical technique and irradiation technology all accounts for the recent progress. For surgery, some of the biopsy and even tumor excision can now be performed under minimal invasive approach with endoscopic method. However, precaution has to be taken that adequate exposure and complete excision is still the goal and first priority for most childhood solid tumors. For irradiation, more precise and accurate ways to delivery irradiation such as intensity modulated radiation therapy (IMRT) or image guided radiation therapy (IGRT or TOMO-RT) can minimize the injury to normal tissues significantly [29, 30].

Brain tumors are the second most common group of childhood cancers. Unlike the adult brain tumors, majority of childhood brain tumors can be cured [31-33]. For example, the most common type of childhood brain tumor is medulloblastoma [34]. With adequate combination of treatment, the long term survival can be above 80% [35]. For astrocytoma, around half of them belong to low grade glioma and they can also be treated with surgery or low intensity chemotherapy nowadays with long progression free survival [36]. The 3rd most common group of brain tumor in Chinese children is germ cell tumor. More than 90% of children with central nervous system germ cell tumor can be cured with chemotherapy plus radiation therapy nowadays [37]. In particularly for dysgerminoma, the most common form of germ cell tumor in childhood, surgical excision is not even required.

In recent years, with the blessing of massive information that we obtained via molecular biology, we understand much more about the pathogenesis and treatment resistant mechanisms of various cancers [38]. Specific therapeutic targets can be identified in many cancers and as a consequence, targeted therapeutic agents in the form of either small molecules or monoclonal antibodies have been developed in an exponential manner [39, 40]. Unfortunately, most of these agents are designed for adult cancers and due to the relatively small market share of childhood cancers, the development of childhood cancers specific targeted therapy is lagging behind. Some of these targeted therapy originally designed for adult cancers can also apply to a small group of childhood cancer patients. That includes the tyrosine kinase inhibitor imatinib for the treatment of chronic myeloid leukemia and Philadelphia chromosome positive ALL [41]. One of the few exceptions is the anti-ganglioside-2 (anti-GD2) monoclonal antibody designed for childhood neurobalstoma [42, 43]. It has been shown that as a combination therapy with other treatment modalities, anti-GD2 containing regimen can achieve 20 to 30% additional survival advantage in children with metastatic neuroblastoma. Future effort should encourage government funding agencies, scientific and clinical researchers to pay more attention to the development of specific targeted therapeutic agents for childhood cancers.

Despite the apparent optimism that we have for the treatment outcome of childhood cancers, we are still facing with quite a number of long term problems [44-46]. For example, we started to notice that up to 5 to 10% of children who experienced radiation therapy in the past may develop 2nd cancer 10 or 20 years later and the cumulative incidence can be as high as 20% after 30 years [47]. Even with chemotherapy alone, a small proportion of children also develop 2nd cancer in the form of therapy related leukemia or 2nd solid tumor [48]. Chemotherapy, especially cisplatin, can induce hearing impairment in the form high tone deafness [49]. For patients with brain tumor, the disease itself and the cranial irradiation may induce long term neurological damage resulting in physical or mental handicaps [50, 51]. Cranial irradiation can also induce partial or total pituitary dysfunction leading to a spectrum of endocrine and learning abnormalities [50, 52]. Chemotherapy, in particularly adriamycin, can induce long term cardiac toxicity in childhood cancer survivors and predispose them to early heart failure [53-55]. Long term renal dysfunction involves the glomeruli or renal tubules can be caused by cisplatin or ifosphamide administration [56, 57]. Even though these alarming long term complications may occur in childhood cancer survivors, fortunately it is relatively uncommon. But as a precaution, long term follow up of childhood cancer survivors is mandatory in order to identify any of these emerging organ dysfunctions in the early stage [58].

Another area of concern in the field of childhood cancers is pediatric palliative care [59]. Many countries still don't have a comprehensive pediatric palliative care program [60]. Childhood hospice facility is also a rarity in most countries including some developed countries. The end of life or quality of death measurement only includes the adult population. Many of the pediatricians do not have formal pediatric palliative care. The end results are that unnecessary aggressive therapies are often applied up to the very last moment in order to satisfy the wishes of the parents but not the children. Difficult terminal symptoms are often not handled properly due to the usual tattoo and stigma in using some medications such as morphine, anti-diarrhea agents and cough suppressants. Ironically, pediatric palliative is even more important in developing countries due to the larger number of untreated cancer patients. It is a cost effective way to relief the patients and their families from the unnecessary suffering and should be emphasized in future comprehensive pediatric care.

CONCLUSION

In summary, with the advancement of science, we now can understand the pathogenesis of cancer much more than before. Well designed treatment protocols and new treatment modalities also drastically improved the outcome. Most children with cancers are no longer incurable nowadays. With multidisciplinary approaches, respectable prognosis is expected. But a significant number of cancer survivors may have residual or late morbidity and requires long term follow-up monitoring. For a small proportion of children with incurable cancers, pediatric palliative care should be provided to make the patients and their families sailing through the end of life journey with less suffering.

REFERENCES

[1] Kaatsch P. Epidemiology of childhood cancer. *Cancer. Treat. Rev.* 2011;36:277-85.

[2] Stiller C. Epidemiology of cancer in adolescents. *Med. Pediatr. Oncol.* 2002;39:149-55.

[3] Baade PD, Youlden DR, Valery PC, et al. Population-based survival estimates for childhood cancer in Australia during the period 1997-2006. *Br. J. Cancer* 2011;103:1663-70.

[4] Guyer B, MacDorman MF, Martin JA, Peters KD, Strobino DM. Annual summary of vital statistics-1997. *Pediatrics* 1998;102:1333-49.

[5] Strahm B, Malkin D. Hereditary cancer predisposition in children: genetic basis and clinical implications. Int J Cancer 2006;119:2001-6.

[6] Stiller CA. Epidemiology and genetics of childhood cancer. *Oncogene* 2004;23:6429-44.

[7] Chene A, Donati D, Orem J, et al. Endemic Burkitt's lymphoma as a polymicrobial disease: new insights on the interaction between Plasmodium falciparum and Epstein-Barr virus. *Semin. Cancer Biol.* 2009;19:411-20.

[8] Huang X, Nolte I, Gao Z, et al. Epidemiology of classical Hodgkin lymphoma and its association with Epstein Barr virus in Northern China. *PLoS One* 2011;6:e21152.

[9] da Silva SR, de Oliveira DE. HIV, EBV and KSHV: viral cooperation in the pathogenesis of human malignancies. *Cancer Lett.* 2011;305:175-85.

[10] Tran H, Nourse J, Hall S, Green M, Griffiths L, Gandhi MK. Immunodeficiency-associated lymphomas. *Blood Rev.* 2008;22:261-81.

[11] Chang MH. Cancer prevention by vaccination against hepatitis B. *Recent Results Cancer Res.* 2009;181:85-94.

[12] Greaves M, Buffler PA. Infections in early life and risk of childhood ALL. *Br. J. Cancer* 2009;100:863.

[13] Li CK, Zee B, Lee J, Chik KW, Ha SY, Lee V. Impact of SARS on development of childhood acute lymphoblastic leukaemia. *Leukemia* 2007;21:1353-6.

[14] Nyari TA, Kajtar P, Bartyik K, Thurzo L, McNally R, Parker L. Seasonal variation of childhood acute lymphoblastic leukaemia is different between girls and boys. *Pathol. Oncol. Res.* 2008;14:423-8.

[15] McNally RJ, Eden TO. An infectious aetiology for childhood acute leukaemia: a review of the evidence. *Br. J. Haematol.* 2004;127:243-63.

[16] Wiemels J, Kang M, Greaves M. Backtracking of leukemic clones to birth. *Methods. Mol. Biol.* 2009;538:7-27.

[17] Worch J, Matthay KK, Neuhaus J, Goldsby R, DuBois SG. Ethnic and racial differences in patients with Ewing sarcoma. *Cancer* 2011;116:983-8.

[18] Smith M, Hare ML. An overview of progress in childhood cancer survival. *J. Pediatr. Oncol. Nurs.* 2004;21:160-4.

[19] Simone JV. History of the treatment of childhood ALL: a paradigm for cancer cure. *Best Pract. Res. Clin. Haematol.* 2006;19:353-9.

[20] Pui CH, Campana D, Evans WE. Childhood acute lymphoblastic leukaemia--current status and future perspectives. *Lancet Oncol.* 2001;2:597-607.

[21] Li CK, Chik KW, Ha SY, et al. Improved outcome of acute lymphoblastic leukaemia treated by delayed intensification in Hong Kong children: HKALL97 study. *Hong Kong Med. J.* 2006;12:33-9.

[22] Pui CH, Gajjar AJ, Kane JR, Qaddoumi IA, Pappo AS. Challenging issues in pediatric oncology. *Nat. Rev. Clin. Oncol.* 2011;8:540-9.

[23] Ko EY, Ritchey ML. Current management of Wilms' tumor in children. *J. Pediatr. Urol.* 2009;5:56-65.

[24] Beverly Raney R, Walterhouse DO, Meza JL, et al. Results of the Intergroup Rhabdomyosarcoma Study Group D9602 protocol, using vincristine and dactinomycin with or without cyclophosphamide and radiation therapy, for newly diagnosed patients with low-risk embryonal rhabdomyosarcoma: a report from the Soft Tissue Sarcoma Committee of the Children's Oncology Group. *J. Clin. Oncol.* 2011; 29:1312-8.

[25] Minn AY, Lyden ER, Anderson JR, et al. Early treatment failure in intermediate-risk rhabdomyosarcoma: results from IRS-IV and D9803--a report from the Children's Oncology Group. *J. Clin. Oncol.* 2011;28:4228-32.

[26] Yuan XJ, Chan GC, Chan SK, et al. Treatment outcome of rhabdomyosarcoma in Hong Kong Chinese children. *Hong Kong Med. J.* 2008;14:116-23.

[27] Pinkerton R, Wills RA, Coory MD, Fraser CJ. Survival from haematological malignancy in childhood, adolescence and young adulthood in Australia: is the age-related gap narrowing? *Med. J. Aust.* 2011;193:217-21.

[28] Patte C, Auperin A, Gerrard M, et al. Results of the randomized international FAB/LMB96 trial for intermediate risk B-cell non-Hodgkin

lymphoma in children and adolescents: it is possible to reduce treatment for the early responding patients. *Blood* 2007;109:2773-80.

[29] Robertson PL. Advances in treatment of pediatric brain tumors. *Neuro. Rx.* 2006;3:276-91.

[30] Ding GX, Coffey CW. Radiation dose from kilovoltage cone beam computed tomography in an image-guided radiotherapy procedure. *Int. J. Radiat. Oncol. Biol. Phys.* 2009;73:610-7.

[31] Reddy AT. Advances in biology and treatment of childhood brain tumors. *Curr. Neurol. Neurosci. Rep.* 2001;1:137-43.

[32] Packer RJ. Childhood brain tumors: accomplishments and ongoing challenges. *J. Child. Neurol.* 2008;23:1122-7.

[33] Kohler BA, Ward E, McCarthy BJ, et al. Annual report to the nation on the status of cancer, 1975-2007, featuring tumors of the brain and other nervous system. *J. Natl. Cancer Inst.* 2011;103:714-36.

[34] Massimino M, Giangaspero F, Garre ML, et al. Childhood medulloblastoma. *Crit. Rev. Oncol. Hematol.* 2011;79:65-83.

[35] Packer RJ, Vezina G. Management of and prognosis with medulloblastoma: therapy at a crossroads. *Arch. Neurol.* 2008;65:1419-24.

[36] Ronghe M, Hargrave D, Bartels U, et al. Vincristine and carboplatin chemotherapy for unresectable and/or recurrent low-grade astrocytoma of the brainstem. *Pediatr. Blood Cancer* 2011;55:471-7.

[37] Kamoshima Y, Sawamura Y. Update on current standard treatments in central nervous system germ cell tumors. *Curr. Opin. Neurol.* 2011;23:571-5.

[38] Stratton MR. Exploring the genomes of cancer cells: progress and promise. *Science* 2011;331:1553-8.

[39] Van den Eynde M, Baurain JF, Mazzeo F, Machiels JP. Epidermal growth factor receptor targeted therapies for solid tumours. *Acta. Clin. Belg.* 2011;66:10-7.

[40] Berz D, Wanebo H. Targeting the growth factors and angiogenesis pathways: small molecules in solid tumors. *J. Surg. Oncol.* 2011;103:574-86.

[41] Fullmer A, Kantarjian H, Cortes J, Jabbour E. New developments in the treatment of chronic myeloid leukemia and Philadelphia-positive acute lymphoblastic leukemia. *Leuk Lymphoma* 2011;52 Suppl 1:81-91.

[42] Yu AL, Gilman AL, Ozkaynak MF, et al. Anti-GD2 antibody with GM-CSF, interleukin-2, and isotretinoin for neuroblastoma. *N. Engl. J. Med.* 2011;363:1324-34.

[43] Cheung NK, Kushner BH, LaQuaglia M, et al. N7: a novel multi-modality therapy of high risk neuroblastoma (NB) in children diagnosed over 1 year of age. *Med. Pediatr. Oncol.* 2001;36:227-30.

[44] Haddy RI, Haddy TB. Lifetime follow-up care after childhood cancer. *J. Am. Board. Fam. Med.* 2011;23:647-54.

[45] Robison LL, Armstrong GT, Boice JD, et al. The Childhood Cancer Survivor Study: a National Cancer Institute-supported resource for outcome and intervention research. *J. Clin. Oncol.* 2009;27:2308-18.

[46] Mertens AC. Cause of mortality in 5-year survivors of childhood cancer. *Pediatr. Blood. Cancer* 2007;48:723-6.

[47] Friedman DL, Whitton J, Leisenring W, et al. Subsequent neoplasms in 5-year survivors of childhood cancer: the Childhood Cancer Survivor Study. *J. Natl. Cancer Inst.* 2011;102:1083-95.

[48] Varan A, Kebudi R. Secondary malignant neoplasms after childhood cancer. *Pediatr. Hematol. Oncol.* 2011;28:345-53.

[49] Rybak LP, Whitworth CA, Mukherjea D, Ramkumar V. Mechanisms of cisplatin-induced ototoxicity and prevention. *Hear. Res.* 2007;226:157-67.

[50] Mulhern RK, Merchant TE, Gajjar A, Reddick WE, Kun LE. Late neurocognitive sequelae in survivors of brain tumours in childhood. *Lancet Oncol*. 2004;5:399-408.

[51] Khong PL, Leung LH, Fung AS, et al. White matter anisotropy in post-treatment childhood cancer survivors: preliminary evidence of association with neurocognitive function. *J. Clin. Oncol.* 2006;24:884-90.

[52] Peckham VC. Learning disabilities in long-term survivors of childhood cancer: concerns for parents and teachers. *Int. Disabil. Stud.* 1991;13:141-5.

[53] Speyer J, Wasserheit C. Strategies for reduction of anthracycline cardiac toxicity. *Semin. Oncol.* 1998;25:525-37.

[54] Cheung YF, Li SN, Chan GC, Wong SJ, Ha SY. Left ventricular twisting and untwisting motion in childhood cancer survivors. *Echocardiography* 2011;28:738-45.

[55] Cheung YF, Hong WJ, Chan GC, Wong SJ, Ha SY. Left ventricular myocardial deformation and mechanical dyssynchrony in children with normal ventricular shortening fraction after anthracycline therapy. *Heart* 2011;96:1137-41.

[56] Skinner R. Chronic ifosfamide nephrotoxicity in children. *Med. Pediatr. Oncol.* 2003;41:190-7.

[57] Rossi R, Kleta R, Ehrich JH. Renal involvement in children with malignancies. *Pediatr. Nephrol.* 1999;13:153-62.

[58] Leisenring WM, Mertens AC, Armstrong GT, et al. Pediatric cancer survivorship research: experience of the Childhood Cancer Survivor Study. *J. Clin. Oncol.* 2009;27:2319-27.

[59] Pritchard S, Cuvelier G, Harlos M, Barr R. Palliative care in adolescents and young adults with cancer. *Cancer* 2011;117:2323-8.

[60] Wolfe J. Recognizing a global need for high quality pediatric palliative care. *Pediatr. Blood Cancer* 2011;57:187-8.

In: Pediatric Cancer
Editor: William Li
ISBN: 978-1-61942-112-7

Chapter 2

THE IMPACT OF CANCER ON THE PSYCHOSOCIAL WELL-BEING AND QUALITY OF LIFE OF HONG KONG CHINESE CHILDREN

William H. C. Li
School of Nursings, Li Ka Shing Faculty of Medicine
The University of Hong Kong, Hong Kong S.A.R., China

ABSTRACT

The diagnosis and treatment of cancer can be a stressful and threatening experience, particularly for children. Although survival rates are higher than ever as a result of new technology and breakthroughs in cancer treatment, the course of treatment for cancer is still a very stressful experience in the life of a child. Unfortunately, most research in childhood cancer has traditionally concentrated on medical issues, and has disregarded the importance of the emotional and psychosocial well-being of children with cancer. Furthermore, most studies of childhood cancer conducted in Hong Kong have focused on examining the psychological well-being and quality of life of family members or caregivers. A review of the literature reveals that so far very few studies have attempted to investigate the experience of cancer from children's own perspectives in Hong Kong Chinese context. The aim of this chapter is to shed light on the psychosocial well-being and quality of life in Hong

Kong Chinese children hospitalized with cancer based on the findings of two recent studies.

Study One: The objective of Study One was to examine the impact of cancer on Hong Kong Chinese children's physical, emotional, and psychosocial well-being. A cross-sectional study was employed. Ninety-eight Hong Kong Chinese children aged 7 to 15 years, admitted for treatment of cancer in 2 paediatric oncology units of 2 different hospitals, were invited to participate in the study. Participants were asked to respond to the Chinese version of the State Anxiety Scale and the Center for Epidemiologic Studies Depression Scale for Children during hospitalization. Besides, a brief semi-structured interview was conducted with each participant before discharge home.

Study Two: The objective of study two was to explore the relationships among treatment-related symptoms, depressive symptoms and quality of life of Chinese children hospitalized with cancer. A cross-sectional study was employed. One hundred and thirty-five Hong Kong Chinese children aged 9 to 16 years, admitted for treatment of cancer in a paediatric oncology unit, were invited to participate in the study. Participants were asked to respond to the Chinese version of the Center for Epidemiologic Studies Depression Scale for Children (CES-DC) and the Chinese version of the Pediatric Quality of Life Inventory TM (PedsQL TM) Cancer Module. Additionally, each participant was asked to report the number and severity of the treatment-related symptoms that they experienced.

The results of Study One showed that children reported considerably high state anxiety scores on admission for treatment of cancer. Besides, semi-structured interviews revealed that nearly all children expressed different degrees of sadness and worry. Additionally, findings from this study indicated that more than half of the participants were potentially at risk for depression, or at least presented some depressive symptoms during their stay in the hospital. The results of Study Two indicated that there were high correlations between treatment-related symptoms and quality of life, treatment-related symptoms and depressive symptoms, and depressive symptoms and quality of life, with children reporting greater symptom severity experiencing higher levels of depression and a lower level of quality of life.

These two studies have addressed a gap in the literature by investigating the experience of cancer, in particular the quality of life from children's own perspectives in Hong Kong Chinese context. The results reveal that cancer has tremendous impact on children's physical, emotional, psychosocial well-being and quality of life. There is an imperative need for nurses to evaluate appropriate nursing interventions that can help children ease the burden of cancer treatment, enhance their quality of life and provide support for them to fight cancer at every step of their long and difficult journey.

INTRODUCTION

Childhood cancer is the second leading cause of death among Hong Kong children above the age of one, next only to accident and poisoning, which claims the lives of 50-60 children a year (Children's Cancer Foundation, 2011). There are approximately 150 newly diagnosed cases of childhood cancer each year, and the incidence of childhood cancer is about 10 per 100,000 children (Hong Kong Cancer Registry, 2009). Similar to Western countries, the most common types of childhood cancer are leukemia, Germ-cell and gonadal tumours, brain tumour and lymphoma (Wills, 2009; Yin and Twinn, 2004).

Recent advances in cancer screening and treatment have resulted in a decrease in mortality rates (Li, Chung, and Chiu, 2010; Stam, Grootenhuis, Caron, and Last, 2006). According to the Children's Cancer Foundation (http://www.ccf.org.hk/), the chance of a cure for most types of leukemia is about 70%, and more than 80% of children with lymphoma are curved. However, despite the improved prognosis, the course of cancer treatment continues to be a very stressful and distressing experience in the life of a child (Stam et al., 2006). Treatment of cancer incorporates chemotherapy, radiotherapy, surgery and bone marrow transplantation, alone or in combination, any or all of which may lead to long-term and lasting physical and psychosocial damage (Dowling and Hockenberry, 2003; Enskar and von Essen, 2008). Most children enter hospital not only for treatment of cancer but also of complications and side effects, such as fever, infections, stomatitis, anaemia, bleeding, and nausea and vomiting. Additionally, children are more vulnerable to the stress of illness than adults because their limited cognitive capacities, lack of self-control and greater dependence on others (Li, Lopez, and Lee, 2007). Children's inability to understand the reasons for their illness and medical treatment can add to their anxiety, fear, anger, uncertainty and feeling of helplessness (Li et al., 2007). Therefore, the consequences of cancer may severely affect a child's quality of life (Langeveld, Grootenhuis, Voute, Haan, and Bos, 2004; Savage, Riordan, and Hughes, 2009).

As increasing numbers of children are being cured of the physiological aspects of cancer, there is a growing awareness of the importance of their psychosocial well-being and quality of life. Indeed, ensuring healthy physical and psychosocial well-being in children hospitalized with cancer, in particular enhancing their quality of life should be a prime concern of healthcare professionals (Bradwell, 2009). It is crucial thus for healthcare professionals to develop and evaluate appropriate interventions with the aim of promoting physical and psychosocial well-being for children with cancer and enhancing their quality of life. Before this can be achieved, the impact of cancer and its treatment on children's physical and psychosocial well-being, in particular their quality of life must be fully understood. The National Cancer Institute in the United States (http://www.cancer.gov/) has emphasized the importance of assessing and evaluating patients' quality of life to gain a better understanding of the impact of cancer and its treatment from the patient's perspective. Nevertheless, whilst much of the research has concentrated on medical issues or treatment outcomes, the impact of cancer and the side effects of treatment on children's quality of life remain relatively underexplored. Some Western studies have investigated the experience of cancer from children's own perspectives (Hedström, Haglund, Skolin, and Essen, 2003; Penkman, Scott-Lane, and Pelletier, 2006). However, most studies of childhood cancer in Hong Kong have focused on examining the experience, psychological well-being and quality of life of family members or caregivers (Wills, 2009; Wong, and Chan, 2006; Yiu, and Twinn, 2001). A review of the literature reveals that so far very few studies have attempted to investigate the experience of cancer from a child's own perspective in the Hong Kong Chinese context.

Conversely, a comprehensive review of the mental health of children reveals that there are differences in the cognitive behaviour of Hong Kong Chinese children when compared with their Western counterparts (Wong and Tsoi, 1999). Hong Kong Chinese children are more submissive, and generally lack creativity, and creative thinking when compared with Western children. This may be the result of Hong Kong's socio-cultural emphasis on obedience and social conformity, academic performance, inhibition of self-expression, and avoidance of being deviant or making mistakes (Tsoi and Pryde, 1999). A recent longitudinal study to examine the relationships between perceived parental psychological control and psychological well-being in Hong Kong Chinese children revealed that parental psychological control may inhibit the development of positive mental well-being and affect emotional life in children (Shek, 2007). On the other hand, it is well documented that Chinese culture is deeply influenced by the philosophical concepts of Confucianism (Chan, Cheung, Mok, Cheung, andTong, 2006) and that this philosophy is reflected in certain notions of fatalism among Chinese people with respect to healthcare. They tend to believe that there is very little that can be done to change their fate, and therefore seem to think that life-threatening diseases such as cancer cannot be prevented (Li, 2009). Because the cultural context in which they live is drastically different from that of Western children, the way that Chinese children view the nature and meaning of their illness will also differ considerably from those of Western children. Consequently, it is uncertain whether the impact of cancer on Chinese children is similar to that experienced by children in the West. Given these issues, the aim of this paper is to shed light on the impact of cancer on the physical and psychosocial well-being, in particular the quality of life of Hong Kong Chinese children hospitalized with cancer based on the findings of two recent studies.

METHOD: STUDY ONE

The aim of the study one was to examine the impact of cancer on physical, emotional, and psychosocial well-being of Hong Kong Chinese children hospitalized with cancer.

Design and Sample

A cross-sectional study was employed in 2008. Hong Kong Chinese children admitted for treatment of cancer in 2 paediatric oncology units of two acute public hospitals, meeting the inclusion criteria for the study, were invited to participate in the study. The inclusion criteria were: (1) all children should be aged 7 to 15 years, (2) children should be able to speak Cantonese and read Chinese, and (3) children should be diagnosed with cancer within the previous 6 months and undergoing active medical treatment. We excluded children with cognitive and learning problems identified from their medical records. A total of 98 children hospitalized with cancer were recruited during a 10-month period.

Study Procedures

Approval for the study was obtained from the hospital ethics committee. Written consent was obtained from the parents after they were told the purposes of the study. Each child was also invited to put his/her name on a special children's consent form. The children and their parents were informed that they had the right to withdraw from the study at any time and were assured of the confidentiality of the study.

On admission to the oncology units, demographic data of children and their parents were collected by research nurse using the demographic form.

Children were then asked to respond to the short form of the Chinese version of the State Anxiety Scale for Children (CSAS-C). On day 7 after admission or upon discharge, children were asked to respond to the Chinese version of the Center for Epidemiologic Studies Depression Scale for Children (CES-DC). Shortly after, a short interview was conducted with each child. The interview for each child lasted approximately 10 minutes. The interviews were semi-structured and audio-taped. An interview guide was used and questions asked were as follows: Can you tell me your experience or feeling when you were diagnosed with cancer? How has the cancer, in particular during the course of treatment, affected your physical and psychosocial well-being? As young children might have limited verbal and cognitive capacities to express themselves and would be perplexed by the open-ended questions, only children aged 8 to 15 years were invited for the interview.

RESULTS: STUDY ONE

The results of this study revealed that children most often viewed pain resulting from diagnostic procedures and treatments as one of the worst aspects of their cancers. Moreover, nausea, lack of appetite and fatigue were the most common physical concerns reported by children hospitalized with cancer. As for the impact of cancer on the on the emotions, results indicate that most children have considerably high state anxiety scores on admission for treatment for cancer.

The results of semi-structured interviews also revealed that nearly all children expressed different degrees of sadness and worry. Owing to the diagnosis of cancer was often so unexpected, some children reported that they were feeling "shock" when they were told of the diagnosis. Findings from this study also indicated that more than half the participants were potentially at risk of depression, or at least presented some depressive symptoms during their stay in hospital.

As for the impact of cancer on psychosocial well-being, the issues most frequently talked about by children in the interviews were confinement and feeling of alienation. Furthermore, a change in appearance, in particular hair loss, was a major concern for older children, which affected their psychosocial well-being.

METHOD: STUDY TWO

The aim of study two was to explore the relationships among treatment-related symptoms, depressive symptoms and quality of life in Chinese children hospitalized with cancer.

Design and Sample

A cross-sectional study was employed in one of the largest acute-care hospitals in Hong Kong with a well-established paediatric oncology unit. Hong Kong Chinese children admitted for treatment of cancer, meeting the inclusion criteria for the study, were invited to participate in the study. The inclusion criteria were: (1) all children should be aged 9 to 16 years, (2) children should be able to speak Cantonese and read Chinese, and (3) children should be diagnosed with cancer within the previous 6 months and undergoing active treatment. We excluded children with cognitive and learning problems identified from their medical records. It is understandable that younger children may well be more vulnerable to the sequela of cancer treatment, but those younger children may have limited verbal and cognitive capacities in expressing themselves and be perplexed by the questionnaires. For this reason, only children aged 9-16 years were invited to participate in the study. A total of 135 children hospitalized with cancer were recruited during a 15-month period from 2010 to 2011.

Study Procedures

Approval for the study was obtained from the hospital ethics committees. Written consent was obtained from the parents after they were told the purpose of the study. They were given the option to participate or refuse their child's involvement in the study. The children were also invited to put their names on a special children's assent form and told that their participation was voluntary.

Data were collected in a paediatric oncology ward. Demographic data of children and their parents were collected by research nurse using the demographic form on day 4 after admission. On day 4 after admission, cancer treatment should be normally started. After recording of demographic data, all participants were asked to respond to the Chinese version of the Center for Epidemiologic Studies Depression Scale for Children (CES-DC) and the

Chinese version of the Pediatric Quality of Life Inventory ™ (PedsQL™) Cancer Module. Additionally, each participant was asked to report the number and severity of the treatment-related symptoms that they experienced. The severity of the symptoms were rated on a 5-point scale of 0 (none) to 4 (very severe). All the participants were able to give direct, full responses to these assessment tools without meeting any difficulty.

RESULTS: STUDY TWO

The results showed that of 135 participants, most of them had been diagnosed with leukaemia and lymphoma. Most participants (64.4%) received chemotherapy to treat their cancer, with around 24% receiving more than one treatment. The results revealed that hair loss, nausea and vomiting, loss of appetite, feeling sluggish, pain and fever were the most common treatment-related symptoms reported by these children, very similar to a previous study (Study One) conducted in a Hong Kong Chinese context. As to the type of treatment received, the results showed that of three single types (surgery, chemotherapy and radiotherapy) participants receiving chemotherapy reported greater severity of symptoms. However, results indicated that participants receiving combined treatment generally experienced greater severity of symptoms than those participants receiving single type of treatment. This is understandable, as every cancer treatment has unique and similar side effects on physiological well-being, and children receiving more than one treatment might well experience more, and more severe, treatment-related symptoms. Among all types of cancer treatment, results indicated that children receiving chemotherapy plus radiotherapy suffered significantly greater severity of treatment-related symptoms and symptomatology of depression, and lower levels of quality of life.

The results of this study revealed that more than half of the participants scored at or above the cut-off scores of 16, indicating that, at least they presented some depressive symptoms as measured by the CES-DC. The findings are consistent with Study One, showing that children hospitalized with cancer are potentially at risk for depression. Conversely, the results of the present study revealed that there were high correlations between treatment-related symptoms and quality of life, treatment-related symptoms and depressive symptoms, and depressive symptoms and quality of life, with children reporting greater symptom severity experiencing higher levels of depression and a lower level of quality of life.

A multiple regression analysis was performed to examine whether treatment-related and depressive symptoms can predict the health-related quality of life of children hospitalized with cancer, after controlling for the possible effects of age, gender, diagnosis and type of treatment. The results indicated that treatment-relative symptoms formed a comparatively strong predictor of health-related quality of life.

DISCUSSION

Research indicates that increased cancer survival rates are accompanied by an increase in associated physiological and psychosocial problems. Whilst much of the attention has focused on the medical treatment and prognosis, the consequences of cancer and its treatments on psychosocial well-being and quality of life of children hospitalized with cancer remain relatively underexplored. Based on the findings of the two recent studies conducted in Hong Kong Chinese context, the aim of this paper was to explore examine the impact of cancer on Hong Kong Chinese children's physical and psychosocial well-being. In particular, emphasis is placed on the exploration of how cancer and its treatment affect the quality of life of these children.

The results of both studies (Study One and Two) revealed that more than half of the participants were potentially at risk of depression, or at least presented some depressive symptoms as measured by the CES-DC. In comparison with previous studies (Li, Chung, and Ho, 2010; Li, Chan, Chung, and Chui, 2010) using the same scale to measure depressive symptoms of a similar age group of Hong Kong Chinese schoolchildren without cancer, the results revealed that the mean depressive symptom scores for children hospitalized with cancer were found to be relatively higher than those schoolchildren without cancer. Although it cannot be assumed from these cross-sectional studies that there is a high risk of depression for children with cancer, many previous studies conducted in Western countries have revealed that children with cancer are at high risk of depression (Cavusoglu, 2001; Dejong and Fombonne, 2006; Matziou, Perdikaris, Galanis, Dousis, and Tzoumakas, 2008). The results of Study Two also indicated that greater symptomatology of depression in children with cancer is associated with poorer quality of life. Additionally, there is some evidence that depressive symptoms predict suicidal tendencies (Ell, Sanchez, and Vourlekis, 2005; Stewart, Lam, Betson, and Chung, 1999). Previous research also has also shown that survivors of childhood cancer are at an elevated risk for suicidal tendencies, even many years after treatment (Recklitis, Lockwood, Rothwell, and Diller, 2006). For these reasons, the presentation of depressive symptoms in children hospitalized with cancer cannot be overlooked or underestimated.

The semi-structured interview conducted in Study One showed that quite a number of children hospitalized with cancer, in particular the older children, were anxious about their academic performance as a result of suspension from school, which was seldom reported in Western literature. One possible reason is that the cultural context in Hong Kong is one where Chinese parents place a considerable emphasis on academic performance and they regard academic achievements as the top priority in child care. Given this cultural context, Hong Kong Chinese children are under tremendous pressure to excel in academic performance. Unlike some Western countries, Hong Kong does not have law to support the educational opportunity for the hospitalized children. Although some hospital teachers from Hong Kong Red Cross (voluntary organization) are available to provide bedside teaching to help sick children regain academic progress during periods of hospitalization, such teachers could only meet with hospitalized children 2-3 times a week due to limited resources.

The Study One did not measure directly the quality of life in children hospitalized with cancer, instead of examining their physical, emotional and psychosocial well-being. Nevertheless, the World Health Organization (1948) defined health as complete physical, mental and social well-being and not merely the absence of disease. This concept has evolved to quality of life, which includes physical, psychological and social components (Varni, Burwinkle, Katz, Meeske, and Dickinson, 2002). Therefore, the results of Study One could actually reflect the quality of life of children hospitalized with cancer.

On the other hand, the Study Two directly assessed the quality of life of children hospitalized with cancer using the Pediatric Quality of Life Inventory ™ (PedsQL™) Cancer Module. The PedsQL™ Cancer Module is a disease-specific instrument developed to capture the multidimensional construct of the health-related quality of life (HRQOL) among paediatric patients with cancer, which includes physical, psychological and social functioning dimensions (Varni, Burwinkle, Katz, Meeske, and Dickinson, 2002). The results revealed that there was a high negative correlation between treatment-related symptoms and quality of life, with children reporting greater symptom severity experiencing lower level of quality of life. The findings are consistent with previous studies from the West, showing that greater symptom severity is associated with poor psychosocial well-being and quality of life (Williams, Schmideskamp, Ridder, and Williams, 2006).

Implication for Practice

The findings of these two studies have important implications for practice. First, both studies found that a significant number of children presented depressive symptoms during the course of cancer treatment in hospital. For children with cancer, feeling depressed may not only severely affect their quality of life, but may even be detrimental to their physical and psychological health (Cavusoglu, 2001). Therefore, it is crucial for nurses working in paediatric oncology units to recognize signs and symptoms of depression in children hospitalized with cancer at an early point, and subsequently take appropriate interventional steps to promote their psychosocial well-being so as to enhance their positive adaptation to treatment and hospitalization. Second, the results of Study Two indicated that children receiving combined treatment generally experienced greater severity of symptoms. Specifically, results showed that children receiving chemotherapy plus radiotherapy suffered significantly greater severity of treatment-related symptoms and symptomatology of depression, and lower levels of quality of life. It is therefore essential for health care professionals to pay more attention to those children receiving combined cancer treatment, in particular for those receiving chemotherapy plus radiotherapy. Third, results of Study Two revealed that there was a high negative correlation between the treatment-related symptoms and qualify of life, with children reporting greater symptom severity experiencing lower level of quality of life. Therefore, the presentation of treatment-related symptoms in children hospitalized with cancer cannot be overlooked or underestimated. Indeed, ensuring healthy psychosocial well-being in children hospitalized with cancer, in particular enhancing their quality of life should be a prime concern of healthcare professionals. Health care professionals should not only concentrated on medical issues or treatment outcomes, there is an imperative needs for them to develop and evaluate interventions that can promote the psychosocial well-being of such children and help them maintain a good quality of life. Last but not least, the study revealed that treatment-related symptoms are a strong predictor of quality of life of children hospitalized with cancer, and may be a useful indicator for screening those children who are likely to exhibit psychosocial distress or are at high risk of depression. Most importantly, it is crucial for nurses to be sensitive and knowledgeable about the treatment-related symptoms of cancer treatment and its effects on children's psychosocial well-being and quality of life. Understanding these treatment-related symptoms may help nurses to develop appropriate and effective interventions with the aims of alleviating symptom severity, and thus promoting the child's psychosocial well-being and quality of life.

Limitation of the Studies

The use of convenience sampling limits the ability of these studies to generalize the results. Another limitation is that these two studies rely mainly on self-reporting instruments and interviews to document children's physical and psychosocial well-being, and quality of life. It is recommended that future studies should also obtain information from parents' perspective on the physical and psychosocial well-being of their children. Information from parents may further enhance our understanding of the impact of cancer and its treatments on the quality of life of children. Additionally, younger children, such as aged less than 7 were not included in these two studies. It is understandable that younger children may have limited verbal and cognitive capacities in expressing themselves and be perplexed by the questionnaires. However, it is believed that younger children may well be more vulnerable to the side effects of cancer treatment. Therefore, future studies may consider using alternative assessment technique such as behavioural observation to document children's behaviour and emotional responses to medical treatment and hospitalization. The advantage of using behavioural observation is that it is not affected by the limited verbal and cognitive capacities of young children.

Conclusion

Despite its possible limitations, these two studies have addressed a gap in the literature by investigating the experience of cancer, in particular the quality of life from children's own perspectives in Hong Kong Chinese context, an area of research that has been underrepresented in the literature. The results reveal that cancer and its treatment have tremendous impact on children's physical, emotional, psychosocial well-being and quality of life. There is an imperative need for nurses to evaluate appropriate interventions that can help children ease the burden of cancer treatment, enhance their quality of life and provide support for them to fight cancer at every step of their long and difficult journey. Most importantly, it is crucial to empower them develop a positive view of the impact that the cancer experience has upon their lives.

REFERENCES

Bradwell, M. (2009). Survivors of childhood cancer. *Pediatric Nursing, 21*(4), 21-24.

Cavusoglu, H. (2001). Depression in children with cancer. *Journal of Pediatric Nursing, 16*(5), 380-385.

Chan, E. A., Cheung, K., Mok, E., Cheung, S., and Tong, E. (2006). A narrative inquiry into the Hong Kong Chinese adults' concepts of health through their cultural stories. *International Journal of Nursing Studies,43*(3), 301-309.

Children's Cancer Foundation. Publications: Leaflets. Cancer in Children. http://www.ccf.org.hk/leaflet/all3.htm. Accessed March 8, 2011.

Dejong, M., Fombonne, E. (2006). Depression in paediatric cancer: An overview. *Psycho-Oncology, 15*, 553-566.

Dowling, J. S., and Hockenberry, M. (2003). Sense of humor, childhood cancer stressors, and outcomes of psychosocial adjustment, immune function, and infection. *Journal of Pediatric Oncology Nursing*, 20, 271-292.

Ell, k., Sanchez, K., and Vourlekis, B. (2005) Depression, receipt of depression care, and correlates of depression among low-income women with breast or gynecological cancer. *Journal of Clinical Oncology*, 23, 3052-3060.

Enskar, K., von Essen, L. (2008). Physical problems and psychosocial function in children with cancer. *Pediaticr Nursing, 20*(3), 37-41.

Hedström, M., Haglund, K., Skolin, I., Essen, L. V. (2003). Distressing events for children and adolescents with cancer: Child, parent, and nurse perceptions. *Journal of Pediatric Oncology Nursing, 20*(3), 120-132.

Hong Kong Cancer Registry, Hospital Authority (2009). Hong Kong Cancer Stat 2007. http://www3.ha.org.hk/cancereg/e_canstat2007.pdf. Accessed March 8, 2011.

Langeveld, N. E., Grootenhuis, M. A., Voute, P. A., Haan, R. J., and Bos, C. V. D. (2004). Quality of life, self-esteem and worries in young adult survivors of childhood cancer. *Psycho-Oncology, 13*, 867-881.

Li, H. C. W., Chung, O. K. J., and Chiu, S. Y. (2010). The impact of cancer on children's physical, emotional, and psychosocial well-being. *Cancer Nursing,* 33(1), 47-54.

Li, H. C. W., Chung, O. K. J., and Ho, K. Y. E. (2010). Center for Epidemiologic Studies Depression Scale for Children: Psychometric testing of the Chinese version. *Journal of Advanced Nursing, 66*(11), 2582-2591.

Li, H. C. W., Lopez, V., and Lee, T. L. I. (2007). Effects of Preoperative Therapeutic Play on Outcomes of School-age Children Undergoing Day Surgery. *Research in Nursing and Health, 30, 320-332.*

Li, W. H. C. (2009). The Importance of Incorporating Cultural Issues into Nursing Interventions for Chinese Populations. In W.T. Chien (Eds). *Strategies in evaluation of complex health care interventions for people with physical or mental health issues*, New York: Nova Biomedical Book.

Li, W. H. C., Chan, S. L. P., Chung, O. K. J. and Chui, M. L. M. (2010) Relationships among mental health, self-esteem and physical health in Chinese adolescents: an exploratory study. *Journal of Health Psychology,* 15(1), 96-106.

Matziou, V., Perdikaris, P., Galanis, P., Dousis, E., and Tzoumakas, K. (2008). Evaluating depression in a sample of children and adolescents with cancer in Greece. *International Nursing Review,* 55, 314-319.

Penkman, L, Scott-Lane, L, Pelletier, W. A. (2006). psychosocial program for pediatric oncology patients: A pilot study of "The Beaded Journey." *Journal of Psychosocial Oncology, 24*, 103-115.

Recklitis, C. J., Lockwood, R. A., Rothwell, M. A., and Diller, L. R. (2006) Suicidal ideation and attempts in adult survivors of childhood cancer. *Journal of Clinical Oncology,* 24(24), 3852-3857.

Savage, E., Riordan, A. O., and Hughes, M. (2009). Quality of life in children with acute lymphoblastic leukaemia: A systematic review. *European Journal of Oncology Nursing, 13*, 36-48.

Shek, D. T. L. (2007). A longitudinal study of perceived parental psychological control and psychological well-being in Chinese adolescents in Hong Kong. *Journal of Clinical Psychology, 63*(1), 1-22.

Stam, H., Grootenhuis, M. A., Caron, H. N., and Last, B. F. (2006). Quality of life and current coping in young adult survivors of childhood cancer: Positive expectations about the further course of the disease were correlated with better quality of life. *Psycho-Oncology, 15*, 31-43.

Stewart, S. M., Lam, T. H., Betson, C., and Chung, S.F. (1999) Suicide ideation and its relationship to depressed mood in a community sample of adolescents in Hong Kong. *Suicide and Life-Threatening Behavior,* 29, 227-240.

Tsoi, M. M., and Pryde, N. A. (1999). Hong Kong's children: overview and conclusion. In N. A. Pryde and M. M Tsoi (EDS.), *Hong Kong's Children: our past, their future* (pp. 573-647). Hong Kong: Centre of Asian Studies, the University of Hong Kong.

Varni, J. W., Burwinkle, T. M., Katz, E. R., Meeske, K., and Dickinson, P. (2002). The PedsQL™ in pediatric cancer: Reliability and validity of the pediatric quality of life inventory™ generic core scale, multidimensional fatigue scale and cancer module. *Cancer*, 94(7), 2090-2106.

Williams, P., Schmideskamp, J., Ridder, L., and Williams, A. (2006). Symptom monitoring and dependent care during chemotherapy in children. *Cancer Nursing, 29*(3), 188-197.

Wills, B. S. H. (2009). Coping with a child with acute lymphocytic leukemia. *Cancer Nursing, 32*(2), E8-E14.

Wong, C. K., and Tsoi, M. M. (1999). Mental health of Hong Kong Children. In N.A. Pryde and M.M. Tsoi (EDS.), *Hong Kong's Children: our past, their future* (pp. 153-220). Hong Kong: Centre of Asian Studies, the University of Hong Kong.

Wong, Y. F. M., and Chan, W. C. S. (2006). The qualitative experience of Chinese parents with children diagnosed of cancer. *Journal of Clinical Nursing,* 15, 710-717.

World Health Organization (1948). *Constitution of the World Health Organization basic document.* Geneva: World Health Organization.

Yin, L. K., and Twinn, S. (2004). The effect of childhood cancer on Hong Kong Chinese families at different stages of the disease. *Cancer Nursing, 27*(1), 17-24.

Yiu, M. C. J., and Twinn, S. (2001) Determining the needs of Chinese parents during the hospitalization of their child diagnosed with cancer: An exploratory study. *Cancer Nursing,* 24(6), 483-489.

In: Pediatric Cancer
Editor: William Li
ISBN: 978-1-61942-112-7

Chapter 3

EFFECTIVENESS OF THERAPEUTIC PLAY INTERVENTION IN PROMOTING THE PSYCHOSOCIAL WELL-BEING OF CHILDREN HOSPITALIZED WITH CANCER

William H. C. Li
School of Nursing, Li Ka Shing Faculty of Medicine
The University of Hong Kong, Hong Kong S.A.R., China

ABSTRACT

Childhood cancer and its treatment have been described as an extremely stressful and threatening experience, which can be emotionally devastating for children. Although survival rates for childhood cancer are higher than ever before, the course of treatment for cancer, such as chemotherapy, surgery or radiotherapy, is still a very stressful experience in the life of a child. Children with cancer may not only be at risk from adverse medical effects; their psycho-social well being may also be severely affected as a result of the cancer and its therapy. The aims of this study were to examine the effectiveness of therapeutic play using virtual reality computer games, in minimizing anxiety and reducing depressive symptoms in Hong Kong Chinese children hospitalized with cancer. Specifically whether a virtual reality computer game is feasible to be implemented in clinical settings and acceptable to health care providers, children hospitalized with cancer and their parents were the focus.

A non-equivalent control group pretest-posttest, between-subject design was employed. Hong Kong Chinese Children (8-16 years of age), admitted to two paediatric oncology units of two different regional acute public hospitals in Hong Kong during a 16-month period, were invited to participate in the study. Of the 133 children, 72 formed the control group receiving routine information preparation and 61 in the experimental group receiving therapeutic play using virtual reality computer games.

The results showed that children in the experimental group reported statistically significant fewer depressive symptoms than children in the control group on day 7. The results, however, although children in the experimental group had lower mean state anxiety scores than children in the control group on day 7, the differences were not statistically significant.

The study provides empirical evidence to support the effectiveness, feasibility and acceptability of using virtual reality computer games in the psychological preparation of children hospitalized with cancer, thus charting a path towards promoting holistic and quality care. It is anticipated that the findings of this empirical study will promote awareness in nurses and parents that play is a very important part of children's life, and that they need play even when they are ill. Additionally, the findings will contribute to promoting nurses' accountability and responsibility for patient care through evidence-based practice.

INTRODUCTION

It has been well documented that the diagnosis and treatment of cancer can be a stressful and threatening experience for children (Li, Chung, and Chiu, 2010; Penkman, Scott-Lane, and Pelletier, 2006). Children are more vulnerable than adults to the illness and medical treatments because of their limited cognitive capacities, lack of self-control, greater dependence on others, and limited life experience and knowledge of the health care system (Li, Lopez, and Lee, 2007). In addition, children's limited ability to understand the reasons of their illness and treatments can add to their anxiety, fear, anger, and feeling of uncertainty and helplessness (Li and Lopez, 2008). Although a mild to moderate level of anxiety can promote better adjustment and is essential for learning (Janis, 1958), excessive anxiety can be detrimental to children's physical and psychosocial well-being. Empirical evidence shows that excessive anxiety hinders children's ability to cope with medical treatment, affects their physical and psychosocial well-being, and encourages negative and uncooperative behaviour during hospitalization (Becher and Sing, 1997; Li and Lopez, 2008).

With advances in cancer screening and medical treatment, the survival rates for childhood cancer are higher than ever before (Stam, Grootenhuis, Caron, and Last, 2006). According to the Canadian Cancer Society Report on Cancer in Children and Youth in 2008 (http://www.candlelighters.ca/educatorsguide/childhoodcancer.html), the survival rates for most childhood cancers were close to 80%. The incidences, types, and survival rates of childhood cancer in Hong Kong are similar with those in United State and Western countries (Children's Cancer Foundation, 2011). Nevertheless, research indicates that increased survival rates are accompanied by an increase in associated psychosocial problems (Enskar and von Essen, 2008; Penkman et al., 2006). Indeed, the course of treatment for cancer, such as chemotherapy, surgery or radiotherapy, alone or in combination, any or all of which may lead to long-term and lasting physical damage (Dowling and Hockenberry, 2003; Enskar and von Essen, 2008). Moreover, cancer and its treatment may not only adversely affect the physical well-being of children hospitalized with cancer; but their psycho-social well being as well (Penkman et al., 2006). Unfortunately, whilst much of the attention has focused on the physiological care of children with cancer, the consequences of cancer and its treatment on psychosocial well-being and quality of life remain relative underexplored.

In a recent study to examine the impact of cancer on Hong Kong Chinese children's physical, emotional and psychosocial well-being (Li et al., 2010), the results reveal that pain, nausea, lack of appetite and feeling sluggish were the most common physical concerns reported by children hospitalized with cancer. As for the impact of cancer on the emotions, results indicate that most children have considerably high state anxiety scores on admission for treatment for cancer. The results of semi-structured interviews also revealed that nearly all children expressed different degrees of sadness and worry. Findings from this study also indicated that more than half the participants were potentially at risk of depression, or at least presented some depressive symptoms during their stay in hospital. As for the impact of cancer on psychosocial well-being, the issues most frequently talked about by children in the interviews were confinement and feelings of estrangement.

Children with cancer displayed depressive symptoms during hospitalization is not only reported in Hong Kong, but also frequently in Western (Cavusoglu, 2001; Dejong and Fombonne, 2006; Essen, Enskär, Kreuger, Larsson, and Sjödén, 2000). In children with cancer, feeling depressed may be detrimental to physical and psychosocial health (Cavusoglu,

2001; Penkman et al., 2006), cause them to give up hope, and may even affect their compliance with treatment and their quality of life (Sung et al., 2011; Williams, Schmideskamp, Ridder, Williams, 2006). Furthermore, there is some evidence that depressive symptoms predict suicidal tendencies (Ell, Sanchez, and Vourlekis, 2005; Stewart, Lam, Betson, and Chung, 1999). The findings of these studies are alarming and warrant special attention by health care professionals. Indeed, helping children ease the psychological burden of cancer treatment is recognized as one of the most vital responsibilities of a nurse (Chien, Lo, Chen, Chen, Chiang, and Chao, 2003). There is an imperative need for nurses to develop and evaluate appropriate psychological nursing interventions that can minimize children's emotional distress during the course of treatment in hospital. Specifically, it is crucial for nurses to find ways to help children resume normal development and make their cancer journey a less difficult one.

Over the past few decades numerous research studies in children's health care have focused on different interventions in promoting psychological health for children hospitalized with cancer (Dowling et al., 2003; Hicks and Lavender, 2001; Penkman et al., 2006). Among all nursing interventions, the provision of information on physiological care in cancer treatment is the most common nursing practice in pediatric oncology units in Hong Kong. Nevertheless, most nursing interventions are focused on procedural information for parents and children, the psychological needs of children hospitalized with cancer have seldom been taken into consideration. In a study to examine the impact of cancer on Hong Kong Chinese children (Li et al., 2010), the results reveal that children hospitalized with cancer experienced considerably high state anxiety scores, and more than half of them displayed depressive symptoms. The result of the study reveals that there is still room for improvement for such preparation.

During the past decade, there has been an increase in the use of therapeutic play intervention to help children cope with the stress of hospitalization. Therapeutic play is a set of structured activities designed according to psychosocial and cognitive development of children, and health-related issues to prepare children psychologically for hospitalization (LeVieux-Anglin and Sawyer, 1993). The central goal of therapeutic play is to facilitate the emotional and physical well-being of hospitalized children (Vessey and Mahon, 1990). Armstrong (2000) claimed that therapeutic play may not only allow children to gain pleasure, but also may help them act out stressful or threatening experiences when faced with stressful medical procedures and unfamiliar environments.

Types of Therapeutic Play

Vessey and Mahon (1990) further classified three types of therapeutic play as emotional outlet play, physiological play, and instructional play.

a) Emotional Outlet Play is designed to help children act out unpleasant experiences and minimize their negative emotional response that majority of children may encounter during hospitalisation. Emotional outlet play can also be used diagnostically to identify children's concern during hospitalisation.
b) Physiological Play is a set of specially designed activities in which children are encouraged to participate to improve their physical health.
c) Instructional (Preparatory) Play is used to prepare children psychologically for stressful medical procedures or surgery. Imparting selected information to children during preparatory play can give children a sense of control over the threatening events and also help them clarify misconceptions that they held previously.

Numerous studies have described the benefits of therapeutic play in helping children cope with the stress caused by illness and hospitalization. These include:

- enhancing paediatric patients' compliance with the medical treatment (Copper and Blitz, 1985),
- alleviating children's distress associated with surgery (Smallwood, 1988),
- facilitating self-expression and providing a mechanism for developing positive coping mechanisms for children cared in an isolation ward (LeVieux-Anglin and Sawyer, 1993),
- demonstrating more co-operation and showing less anxiety during the lumbar puncture procedures (Mansson, Bjorkhem, and Wiebe, 1993),
- improving social interaction, growth and development for paediatric patients with bone marrow transplant (Kuntz, Adams, Zahr, Killen, Cameron, and Wasson, 1996),
- Minimizing negative emotional behaviours in paediatric patients when undergoing the procedure of blood sample collection (Ribeiro, Sabates, and Ribeiro, 2001),

- Identifying the specific psychosocial needs of the paediatric oncology patient (O'Connor and Drennan, 2003) and decreasing their anxiety when undergoing invasive procedures (Frankenfield, 1996), and
- Establishing trust between paediatric patients and the health care provides during the process of nursing (Pan, Chiu, Shen, and Chen, 2004).

All these case studies described in the literature testify to the usefulness of therapeutic play in a hospital setting. Regretfully, the majority of previous research on therapeutic play was case studies, which based on theories and clinical observations. Although these theory-based recommendations seem practical and reasonable, the effectiveness of therapeutic play has seldom been tested. In a randomized controlled trial to examine the effectiveness of therapeutic play intervention on outcomes of children undergoing day surgery, the results showed that children reported lower state anxiety scores and exhibited fewer instances of negative emotional behaviours in pre- and post-operative periods (Li and Lopez, 2008). However, there is a lack of empirical evidence to determine accurately the clinical effectiveness of therapeutic play, in particular using it to ease the psychological burden of children hospitalized with cancer. A review of the literature reveals that there is so far no published study testing the effects of therapeutic play intervention on minimizing psychological distress for children hospitalized with cancer in Hong Kong Chinese context.

As play has traditionally been viewed as less important for hospitalized children by many Chinese parents and some health care professionals when compared with physiological care or medical treatment in Hong Kong (Becher and Sing, 1997), it is not clear whether therapeutic play is an appropriate and acceptable psychological intervention for Chinese children and their parents.

Given the above issues, this study aimed (1) to determine the effectiveness of therapeutic play, using virtual reality computer games, in minimizing anxiety and reducing depressive symptoms in Hong Kong Chinese children hospitalized with cancer, and (2) to examine the feasibility and appropriateness of implementing therapeutic play intervention in Hong Kong clinical settings.

METHOD

Design

The study was carried out in two paediatric oncology units of two different regional acute public hospitals in Hong Kong. The two paediatric oncology units were similar in nature and setting. To examine the effects of therapeutic play intervention, a non-equivalent control group pretest-posttest, between-subject design was employed.

The study was divided into two phases. In phase one, all participants admitted to the oncology unit received usual care (control group). After finishing data collection for the control group, we allowed one month washout period before starting data collection in phase two. All participants admitted to the oncology units in phase two received usual care plus therapeutic play using virtual reality computer games (experimental group)

Sample

Children with cancer admitted to the two paediatric oncology units for treatment of cancer meeting the inclusion criteria for the study, were invited to participate in the study. The inclusion criteria were the following: (1) all children should be aged 8 and 16 years, (2) children should be able to speak Cantonese and read Chinese, and (3) children should be diagnosed with cancer for at least two months and undergoing active medical treatment. The researcher excluded children who with identified cognitive and learning problems in their medical records.

It is understandable that younger children may well be more vulnerable to the side effects of cancer treatment, and thus may benefit from therapeutic play intervention. Yet, those younger than eight may have limited verbal and cognitive capacities in expressing themselves and be perplexed by the questionnaires. For this reason, only children aged 8 to 16 years were invited to participate in the study.

Sample size was calculated to obtained sufficient power to detect differences between the groups. The researcher predicted a medium effect size of differences between two groups based on one prior study (Li and Lopez, 2008) testing the effectiveness of therapeutic play intervention on children's pre- and postoperative anxiety. To predict this effect size of differences between two groups at a 5% significance level ($p < 0.05$) and a power of 0.80,

64 subjects in each group are normally required (Polit and Beck, 2008). The researchers allowed for potential attrition at a rate of 15% for the study, which is common in experimental designs. Accordingly, an addition of 11 participants will be required per group to cover the attrition. Therefore, the total sample size will be 150.

A total of 133 children were recruited during a 16-month period from 2009 to 2010. The response and attrition rates in the control group were 97% and 4% respectively, while those in the experimental group were 85% and 13% respectively. Of the 133 children, 72 formed the control group and 61formed the experimental group.

Intervention

In the control group, children and their parents received routine information preparation from a nurse on physiological care in cancer treatment, such as attention to side effects and complications of cancer treatments, oral hygiene, and nutritional dietary intake.

In the experimental group, apart from receiving usual care, children received approximately thirty minutes therapeutic play intervention, using virtual reality computer games daily (except on Saturday, Sunday and public holidays). The therapeutic play intervention was conducted by a research nurse and implemented in small groups with maximum 4 children in one group in the play area of each oncology unit. Previous studies (Cooper and Blitz, 1985, LeVieux-Anglin and Sawyer, 1993) pointed out that school age children are more peer oriented and they could benefit from group teaching and learning. Moreover, it offers children an opportunity to interact with their peers and creates a non-threatening atmosphere for children to express their concern and fear. To ensure children could be able to participate in the therapeutic play intervention, the time for implementing virtual reality computer games was flexible and repeated sessions were carried out during the daytime. Participants were invited to join the play activities when they were not occupied by any medical treatments or physiological care. The therapeutic play intervention could be terminated if participants complained of tiredness. Before commencing the study, the research nurse received training provided by the Leovation Limited (http://www.leovation.com/) on how to implement the virtual reality computer games. To eliminate the experimenter bias effect, the research nurse responsible for data collection was independent to the research nurse responsible for implementing the therapeutic play intervention to the subjects.

The Content of Therapeutic Play

The content of therapeutic play in this study contained a variety of group playing activities, in particular involves using virtual reality through interactive stimulations created by computer hardware and software to present children with opportunities to engage in environments that appear and feel similar to real-work objects and events. Some activities were more energy-consuming, and some were not. The intervener can, in accordance to children's sex, age, ability, type of disease and general condition, select suitable virtual reality computer games for them to play. Besides, children might also have choice on types of play.

To produce virtual reality environment for children to play, a PlayMotion system was installed in a playroom of the paediatric oncology ward. PlayMotion system is a device that transforms ordinary walls, floors, and ceilings into wildly interactive, virtual playgrounds. It combines the flexibility of video projectors, the computer vision algorithms, and the real time special effects systems of videogames. PlayMotion requires no goggles, gloves, helmets, and markers, and thus making it an immediate, totally intuitive, and completely natural experience. Only the shadows of moving arms are needed to enter exciting, interactive projected play spaces - from flying over a city and creating trance-like waves, ripples and colours to playing football, volleyball or billiards.

The Rationales of Using Virtual Reality Technology in Therapeutic Play

Previous study has showed that virtual reality could provide positive and enjoyable leisure experiences during physical interactions with different game-like virtual environments and potentially lead to increased self-esteem and a sense of self-empowerment for children with physical and intellectual disabilities in clinical settings (Weiss, Bialik, and Kizony, 2003). One advantage of using virtual reality for children to play is that it enables great flexibility in the way it can be interfaced with children and adapted to suit specific therapeutic goals. The child can, in accordance with his or her ability and type of disease, sit or stand while performing within the virtual environment. It is also a real opportunity to provide children with a break from the rigors of hospitalization and treatment as well as a sense of control over their illness and have fun at the same time. Besides, virtual reality provides a platform in which children with illness and unable to perform leisure activities in "real life" settings, may be able to engage in them.

The effectiveness of using virtual reality as an intervention tool in rehabilitation has recently been well-documented (Kizony, Katz, and Weiss, 2003; Schultheis and Rizzo, 2001). There is also some evidence that multi-sensory interactive experiences are an effective method of moving children minds away from anxiety and pain (Steele, Grimmer, Thomas, Mulley, Fulton, and Hoffman, 2003).

Measures

Short-Form of the Chinese Version of the State Anxiety Scale for Children (CSAS-C)

The state anxiety level of participants was measured by using the short form of the CSAS-C. This consists of 10 items, scored from 1 to 3, with total possible scores ranging from 10 to 30. Higher scores indicate greater anxiety. The psychometric properties of the short-form of the CSAS-C have been empirically tested (Li and Lopez, 2007). The results showed that the short-form of the CSAS-C was highly correlated with scores obtained from the full form (r = 0.92), had acceptable internal consistency (r = 0.83), and good convergent validity in differentiating state anxiety of children under stressful and relaxed situations. The results of confirmatory factor analysis further added evidence of the construct validity of the short form of the CSAS-C (Li, Wong, Lopez, 2008).

The Center for Epidemiologic Studies Depression Scale for Children (CES-DC)

Children were assessed for any present of depressive symptoms by use of the CES-DC. The CES-DC was derived from the Center for Epidemiologic Studies Depression Scale for Adult (CES-D) developed by Radloff (1977). The CES-D was then modified to become more child-friendly (Weissman, Orvaschel, and Padian, 1980). The CES-DC comprises 20 fully standardised items to evaluate depressive symptoms. The items consist of short and simple statements in the first person about the emotional, cognitive and behaviour related components of depressiveness. All items are evaluated on a four-point Likert scale in relation to their incidence during the last week, which were scored from 0 to 3 (0 = "not at all," 1 = "a little," 2 = "some," 3 = "a lot"), with total possible scores ranging from 0 to 60, with higher scores indicating greater symptomatology. A score of 16 or greater indicates an individual demonstrating some depressive symptoms (Radloff 1977). The psychometric properties of the CES-DC have been empirically tested (Barkmann, Erhart, and Schulte-Markwort, 2008; Li, Chung, and Ho, 2010), showing adequate internal consistency reliability, good concurrent validity, and excellent construct validity. The results of confirmatory factor analysis showed that there are four factors underlying the CES-DC, which is congruent with hypothesized configuration of the factor structure of the CES-D proposed by Radloff (1977). The four-factor version of the CES-DC is considered to have good factorial validity and stability across age (Barkmann et al., 2008).

Study Procedures

Study approval was obtained from hospital ethics committees. Written consent was obtained from the parents after they were told the purpose of the study. They were given the option to participate or refuse their child's involvement in the study. The children were also invited to put their names on a special children's assent form and told that their participation was voluntary and were assured of the confidentiality of the study.

On admission to the oncology units, demographic data of children and their parents were collected by research nurse using the demographic form. Moreover, baseline state anxiety scores and depressive symptoms of children were assessed. On day 7 after admission or upon discharge, the state anxiety level and depressive symptoms of participants were again assessed.

Data Analysis

The Statistical Package for Social Sciences (SPSS: Version 18.0; SPSS Inc., Chicago, IL, USA) for Windows was used for data analysis. The homogeneity of the experimental and control groups were assessed by using inferential statistics (independent *t*-test and χ^2). Mixed between-within subjects ANOVA (split-plot ANOVA) was used to determine whether therapeutic play, using virtual reality computer games, was more effective in minimizing state anxiety and reducing depressive symptoms of children hospitalized with cancer than that of solely providing routine nursing care during the 1st week of hospitalization.

Null Hypotheses

There will be no statistically significant differences in state anxiety scores in children hospitalized with cancer who receive therapeutic play, using virtual reality computer games or routine information preparation on day 7 after admission or upon discharge.

There will be no statistically significant differences in reporting of depressive symptoms in children hospitalized with cancer who receive therapeutic play, using virtual reality computer games or routine information preparation on day 7 after admission or upon discharge.

RESULTS

Information on the demographic, clinical, and baseline characteristics of the experimental and control groups is presented in Table 1.

The results revealed that the experimental and control groups were similar with respect to the age and gender of children, education attainment of parents, medical diagnosis, and baseline state anxiety scores and depressive symptoms for children, suggesting a high level of homogeneity of variance between these two groups in this study. Almost all participants had been diagnosed with cancer within the previous 12 months, with only three diagnosed more than a year before. The mean and standard deviation of the state anxiety and depressive symptom scores in children across the two time periods is shown in Table 2. Approximately 53% and 58% of the children scored at or above the cut-off score of 16 on admission and on day 7, respectively, indicating that they presented some depressive symptoms as measured by the CES-DC.

Effects of Intervention on State Anxiety of Children

The results of mixed between-within subjects ANOVA (Table 3) indicated that there was a statistically significant main effect for time in the state anxiety scores, suggesting a change in the state anxiety scores of children in both groups across the two time periods. Besides, the results indicated that there was a statistically significant interaction effect, indicating that the changes in the state anxiety scores of children over time depended on the types of intervention given. The results of between-subjects effects showed that there was no statistically significant main effect for intervention, suggesting that there was no difference in children's anxiety scores between the two groups on day 7.

Table 1. Comparison of experimental and control groups on demographic, baseline, and clinical characteristics ($n = 133$)

	n (%)		pa
	Experimental (n = 61)	Control (n = 72)	
Gender of Children			
Male	34 (55.7)	39 (54.2)	0.78 ns
Female	27 (44.3)	33 (45.8)	
Medical Diagnosis			
Leukaemia	26 (42.6)	29 (40.3)	0.69 ns
Lymphoma	14 (22.9)	17 (23.6)	
Brain tumour	5 (8.2)	4 (5.6)	
Germ-cell tumour	9 (14.8)	14 (19.4)	
Osteosarcomas	7 (11.5)	8 (11.1)	
Education attainment (parents)			
Primary	5 (8.2)	6 (8.3)	0.88 ns
Lower secondary	18(29.5)	24 (33.3)	
Upper secondary	32 (52.5)	34 (47.2)	
Tertiary	6 (9.8)	8 (11.2)	
Age of children	10.8 (2.1)	11.9 (2.4)	0.71 ns
Children's state anxiety scores	21.1 (4.9)	21.2 (4.7)	0.95 ns
Children's depressive symptoms scores	22.4 (5. 9)	22.1 (5.6)	0.83 ns

ns: not significant at $p > 0.05$.
a Group comparisons *t*-test for continuous and $\chi 2$ for nominal and categorical variables.

Effect of Intervention on Depressive Symptoms of Children

The results of mixed between-within subjects ANOVA (Table 3) indicated that there was a statistically significant main effect for time in the depressive symptoms scores, suggesting a change in the reporting of depressive symptoms by children in both groups across the two time periods. Besides, the results indicated that there was a statistically significant interaction effect, indicating the changes in reporting of depressive symptoms by children over time depended on the types of intervention given. In addition, the results of between-subjects effects showed that there was a statistically significant main effect for intervention, indicating that children in the experimental group reported statistically significant fewer depressive symptoms than children in the control group on day 7. Using the commonly used guidelines proposed by Cohen (1992), the partial eta squared (0.06) indicates that the effect size for the intervention (therapeutic play using virtual reality computer games) was moderate.

Table 2. The mean state anxiety scores and depressive symptom scores in children across two time periods (*n* = 133)

	Mean (S.D.)		
	Experimental (n = 61)	Control (n = 72)	Total (n = 133)
State anxiety on admission	21.1 (4.9)	21.2 (4.7)	21.2 (4.7)
State anxiety scores on day 7	19.5 (4.7)	21.1 (4.5)	20.4 (4.6)
Depression symptom scores on admission	22.4 (5. 9)	22.1 (5.6)	22.20
Depression symptom scores on day 7	20.7 (5.8)	25.9 (6.1)	23.4 (5.9)

Table 3. The results of SPANOVA on state anxiety and depressive symptom scores in children across two time periods (*n* = 133)

	State Anxiety Scores				Depressive Symptom Scores			
	F-value	*p-value*	Eta Squared	Observed Power	*F-value*	*p-value*	Eta Squared	Observed Power
Main effect for time	33.11	0.00	0.20	0.95	17.19	0.00	0.14	0.93
Interaction effect	28.55	0.00	0.19	0.97	115.81	0.00	0.47	0.98
Main effect for intervention	3.42	0.09	0.05	0.67	6.06	0.02	0.06	0.81

DISCUSSION

Research indicates that the cancer and its treatment have tremendous impact on children's physical, emotional, and psychosocial well-being. Whilst much of the attention has focused on the physiological care of children with cancer, the psychological needs of children hospitalized with cancer have seldom been taken into consideration. The aim of this study was to examine the effectiveness of therapeutic play, using virtual reality computer games, in minimizing anxiety and reducing depressive symptoms in Hong Kong Chinese children hospitalized with cancer.

The use of randomized controlled trial represents the most powerful method for establishing cause-and-effect relationships between variables. However, randomization of subjects to different groups was not possible in this study, because there was a possibility of contamination between the two different treatment groups within the setting, and some participants and particularly parents of children might be concerned or disturbed by experiencing a different form of nursing intervention. Given these issues, an alternative method, quasi-experimental (non-equivalent control group), pretest-posttest between-subject design was employed.

Effect of Therapeutic Play Interventions on the State Anxiety of Children

The results of the study showed that children reported considerably high state anxiety scores on admission for cancer treatment. The results were consistent with a previous study (Li et al., 2010), showing that children hospitalized with cancer experienced different degrees of sadness, unhappiness, and worry. However, there was a slightly reduction in the state anxiety scores of children on day 7, regardless of the type of intervention received by children. This is understandable, as most of the children had undergone stressful and painful medical procedures and treatments on day 7, and their worries and anxiety might have lessened. Another reason for the reduction in anxiety level might be that children gain more sense of self-control over the unfamiliar environment and medical procedures on day 7. According to the theory of cognitive appraisal, stress and coping (Lazarus and Folkman, 1984), the individual's evaluation of the threat is influenced by his/her perception of control over a potential threat. Therefore, it was reasoned that if children believed that they had adequate control over the environment or an upcoming medical procedure, the perception of threat would decrease. Owing to the transitory nature of anxiety, the state anxiety score of a child may vary in intensity, fluctuating from time to time as a result of exposure to different situations. However, although children in the experimental group had lower mean state anxiety scores than children in the control group on day 7, the differences were not statistically significant. One possible explanation lies in the difficulty in determining whether children's state anxiety could be expected to respond to therapeutic play interventions, which had a more precise effect on reducing children's depressive symptom, while state anxiety might be less responsive to such intervention. Nevertheless, when examining the effect size and power of therapeutic play intervention on children's state anxiety scores, we found that the effect size was between small and moderate (Eta squared = 0.05), indicating therapeutic play intervention might well be effective. Additionally, the result of the power analysis was only .67, indicating a high chance of committing a type II error (33%). The results suggest that the relationship between type of intervention and children's state anxiety scores on day 7 might have been affected by the limited sample size. It would therefore be interesting to see if further studies using larger samples could find a significant relationship between therapeutic play intervention and children's state anxiety.

The Effects of Therapeutic Play on Children's Depressive Symptoms Scores

The results showed that most children presented some depressive symptoms during their stay in the hospital. The overall mean depressive symptom scores for children on admission and on day 7 were higher than the cut-off point (16). The findings concurred with the results of a previous local study (Li et al., 2010), showing that children hospitalized with cancer are potentially at risk for depression. The results were also consistent with studies conducted in Western countries (Dejong and Fombonne, 2006, Matziou, Perdikaris, Galanis, Dousis, and Tzoumakas, 2008), adding further evidence that children hospitalized with cancer are at high risk of depression.

The findings suggest that there was a change in the reporting of depressive symptoms by children in both groups across the different time periods. However, changes over the different times were dissimilar between the experimental and control groups. Following the admission to the pediatric oncology units, the mean depressive symptom scores among children in the control group increased, as measured on day 7. Because hospitalization and painful medical procedures are anxiety-provoking events and can be emotionally devastating for children (Li et al., 2010), common emotional responses like worry, fear, and uncertainty are likely to be meticulously reported after admission to hospital. Unlike the CSAS-C, which asked children to indicate the degree to which they are experiencing a particular feeling at the current moment, the CES-DC asked them to rate the frequency of depressive symptoms during the past week. This probably explains why children in the control group reported more depressive symptoms on day 7 than on admission. Nevertheless, in contrast to the control group, children receiving therapeutic play activities, using virtual reality computer games, reported statistically significant fewer depressive symptoms than children in the control group. This concurred with the results of a previous study where implementation of therapeutic play activities was found to be effective in helping children cope with the stress of hospitalization (Li et al., 2007).

Implementing therapeutic play for children with cancer during their hospitalization has particular advantages since serious illness and its accompanying stress and physical restriction interrupt the natural play and socialization which is essential for children's normal growth and development. Moreover, owing to low body resistance and susceptibility to infection, most children have relatively few opportunities to engage in leisure activities.

The lack of opportunity to play often leads to the development of dependent behavioral patterns, learned helplessness, and depression (Weiss et al., 2003). A previous study to investigate the impact of cancer on the psychosocial well-being of children hospitalized with cancer revealed that the issues most frequently talked about by children in the interviews were confinement and feeling of alienation.

Therefore, implementing therapeutic play for children with cancer during their hospitalization can provide more opportunity for children to engage in leisure activities, greater involvement in which can improve children's coping skills, decrease their stress, and eventually link to better psychosocial adjustment to illness and hospitalization.

The Feasibility of Using Virtual Reality Computer Games in Clinical Settings

Implementing therapeutic play intervention with virtual reality computer games may require some extra resources, such as those needed in the short run to purchase necessary equipments. However, this will certainly enhance the hospital's capacity to promote quality health in the long run. Indeed, it only takes about half of an hour a day of a staff nurse's time to provide a creative recreational and psychosocial intervention to make the child's cancer journey a less difficult one. Clearly, it would be economically feasible for the healthcare system to consider and utilize this intervention as part of routine nursing care for children hospitalized with cancer. Additionally, as the PlayMotion system is user-friendly and easy to operate, it is expected that the virtual reality computer games implemented in this study will be quickly learnt by nurses, and will take little effort if used regularly. It thus seems feasible and appropriate to implement such games in clinical settings where children are hospitalized with cancer.

The Acceptability of Using Virtual Reality Computer Games by Children and their Parents

The overall results provide some evidence that therapeutic play using virtual reality computer games is effective and feasible in reducing depressive symptoms in children hospitalized with cancer. However, drawing conclusions from research findings is not the end of evidence-based nursing practice; it is crucial to ensure that the research findings can be put into clinical practice. Most importantly, it is essential to find out whether this innovation is acceptable to children and parents. The results of the study showed that the response rate was comparatively low, but with a higher attrition rate in the experimental group. There are some reasons that might shed light on these issues. First, some children refused to participate in the play activities after receiving chemotherapy. Indeed, feeling sluggish after chemotherapy was one of the most common physical concerns reported by children that prevented them from joining any energy-consuming activities (Whitsett, Gudmundsdottir, Davies, McCarthy, and Friedman, 2008). A child in this study claimed that, "I felt powerlessness after chemotherapy. I even found difficulty in getting out of my bed." Second, there are some misconceptions about therapeutic play interventions among parents. Some parents showed reluctance to let their children join the therapeutic play activities as they thought that resting rather than play was the most appropriate method for their recovery, particularly during the acute phase of cancer treatment. Moreover, for fear of their contracting infectious diseases, some parents did not encourage their children to engage in close social contact with other hospitalized children. In view of these concerns, it is advisable to allow those children who have received chemotherapy to have adequate rest for a day prior to introducing them to the computerized interactive virtual space. Moreover, parents should be informed about the prevention of cross-infection. Most importantly, parents should be made aware of the importance of play in promoting children's normal growth and development.

Implications for Practice and Research

The most important implications for nursing practice from this study relate to the determination of the clinical effectiveness of using virtual reality computer games in reducing depressive symptoms in Hong Kong Chinese children hospitalized with cancer. In addition, this study demonstrated the feasibility of using virtual reality computer games as psychological nursing interventions for children hospitalized with cancer. Most importantly, the findings of this study will heighten the awareness of the importance of integrating play activities as an essential component of holistic and quality nursing care to ease the psychological burden of cancer treatment.

The information from this study will promote awareness in nurses and parents that play is a very important for the normal growth and development of children and they need play even when they are ill. If the practice continues at the study hospital and is also introduced in other hospitals, this improvement may be sustained. There are Chinese children living in many parts of the world other than China, Taiwan, Singapore, and Hong Kong. It may be beneficial for nurses in other parts of the world to implement therapeutic play using virtual reality computer games notwithstanding the differences in nursing practice. However, this study mainly focused on Hong Kong Chinese population. It is recommended that further study should be also carried out in children hospitalized with cancer in different cultural settings. Most importantly, we believe that the findings of this study will not only contribute in promoting nurses' accountability and responsibility for patients' care through evidence-based practice, but will also facilitate the development of more autonomy in the advancement of nursing practice.

Limitations

This study was limited in that all data were collected in one setting, which might limit the ability to generalize the result. Another limitation of this study was related to the recruitment issue. There was an outbreak of human swine influenza (H1N1) in Hong Kong at the time of data collection in phase two. According to the Hong Kong Hospital Authority's policy, all non-medical related activities, including research-related activities including the therapeutic play activities were suspended during this period. Consequently, only 61 subjects were recruited to the experimental group before the policy commenced.

Conclusion

Notwithstanding some potential limitations, the study has addressed a gap in the literature by systematically researching the effects of therapeutic play intervention, using virtual reality computer games, on the outcomes of children hospitalized with cancer. This study provides empirical evidence to support the effectiveness of therapeutic play, using virtual reality computer games, in the psychological preparation of children hospitalized with cancer, thus charting a path towards promoting evidence-based, holistic and quality care.

Indeed, there was a considerable amount of positive feedback from children receiving therapeutic play intervention in the two study hospitals. One of their comments was as follows:

> "I was so sad because of the disease, and the environment around me even made me feel more depressed as the ward was full of medical equipment and sick people. It was really boring to stay in bed all day long without anything to do. I never thought there would be some virtual computer games introduced to the ward. It occupied my time or at least let me forget any unhappy event ahead… I was so relaxed while I was playing."

REFERENCES

Armstrong, T. S. H. (2000). The developing role of play preparation in paediatric anaesthesia. *Paeidatric Anaesthesia*, 10, 1-4.

Barkmann, C., Erhart, M., and Schulte-Markwort, M. (2008). The German version of the Centre for Epidemiological Studies Depression Scale for Children: psychometric evaluation in a population-based survey of 7 to 17 years old children and adolescents – results of the BELLA study. *European Child and Adolescent Psychiatric, 17*, 116-24.

Becher, Y., and Sing, A. W. N. (1997). *A new chapter in paediatric health care: A research report to evaluate hospital play services in Hong Kong.* Hong Kong Playright Children's Playground Association Ltd.

Cavusoglu, H. (2001). Depression in children with cancer. *Journal of Pediatric Nursing,16,* 380-385.

Chien, L. Y., Lo, L. H., Chen C. J., Chen, Y. C., Chiang, C. C, and Chao, Y. M. Y. (2003). Quality of life among primary caregivers of Taiwanese children with brain tumor. *Cancer Nursing, 26*, 305-311.

Children's Cancer Foundation. Publications: Leaflets. Cancer in Children. http://www.ccf.org.hk/leaflet/all3.htm. Accessed April 16, 2011.

Cohen, J. (1992). A power primer. *Psychological Bulletin, 112*, 155-159.

Cooper, S. E., and Blitz, J. T. (1985). A therapeutic play group for hospitalized children with cancer. *Journal of Psychosocial Oncology, 3*, 23-37.

Dejong, M., and Fombonne, E. (2006). Depression in paediatric cancer: An overview. *Psycho-Oncology, 15*, 553-566.

Dowling, J. S., Hockenberry, M., and Gregory, R. L. (2003). Sense of humor, childhood cancer stressors, and outcomes of psychosocial adjustment, immune function, and infection. *Journal of Pediatric Oncology Nursing, 20*, 271-292.

Ell, k., Sanchez, K., and Vourlekis, B. (2005) Depression, receipt of depression care, and correlates of depression among low-income women with breast or gynecological cancer. *Journal of Clinical Oncology*, 23, 3052-3060.

Enskar, K, and von Essen, L. (2008). Physical problems and psychosocial function in children with cancer. *Pediatric Nursing, 20*, 37-41.

Essen, L. V., Enskär, K., Kreuger, A., Larsson, B., and Sjödén, P. O. (2000) Self-esteem, depression and anxiety among Swedish children and adolescents on and off cancer treatment. *Acta Paediatrica,* 89, 229-236.

Frankenfield, P.K. (1996). The power of humor and play as nursing interventions for a child with cancer: A case report. *Journal of Pediatric Oncology Nursing, 13*, 15-20.

Hicks, M. D., and Lavender, R. (2001). Psychosocial practice trends in pediatric oncology. *Journal of Pediatric Oncology Nursing, 18*, 143-153.

Kizony, R., Katz, N., and Weiss, P. L. (2003). Adapting an immersive virtual reality system for rehabilitation. *Journal of Visualization and Computer Animation, 14*, 261-8.

Kuntz, N., Adams, J. A., Zahr, L., Killen, R., Cameron, K., and Wasson, H. (1996). Therapeutic play and bone marrow transplantation. *Journal of Pediatric Nursing, 11*, 359-367.

Lazarus, R. S. (1984). Folkman S. *Stress, appraisal and coping*. New York: Springer.

LeVieux-Anglin L., and Sawyer, E. H. (1993). Incorporating play interventions into nursing care. *Pediatric Nursing, 19*, 459-463.

Li, H. C. W. and Lopez, V. (2007). Development and validation of a short form of the Chinese version of the State Anxiety Scale for Children. *International Journal of Nursing Studies, 44*, 566-573.

Li, H. C. W., and Lopez, V. (2008). Effectiveness and appropriateness of therapeutic play intervention in preparing children for surgery: A randomized controlled trial study. *Journal f or Specialists in Pediatric Nursing, 13*, 63-73.

Li, H. C. W., Chung, O. K. J. and Ho, K. Y. E. (2010) Psychometric Testing of the Chinese version of the Center for Epidemiologic Studies Depression Scale for Children. *Journal of Advanced Nursing,* 66*(11), 2582-2591.*

Li, H. C. W., Chung, O. K. J., and Chiu, S. Y. (2010). The impact of cancer on children's physical, emotional, and psychosocial well-being. *Cancer Nursing, 33*(1), 47-54.

Li, H. C. W., Lopez, V. and Lee, T. L. I. (2007). Effects of Preoperative Therapeutic Play on Outcomes of School-age Children Undergoing Day Surgery. *Research in Nursing and Health, 30,* 320-332.

Li, W. H. C., Wong, E. M. L. and Lopez, V. (2008). Factorial structure of the Chinese version of the State Anxiety Scale for Children (short form). *Journal of Clinical Nursing, 17*(13), 1762-1770.

Mansson, M., Bjorkhem, G., and Wiebe, T. (1993). The effect of preparation for lumbar puncture on children undergoing chemotherapy. *Oncology Nursing Forum, 20*, 39-45.

Matziou, V., Perdikaris, P., Galanis, P., Dousis, E., and Tzoumakas, K. (2008). Evaluating depression in a sample of children and adolescents with cancer in Greece. *International Nursing Review, 55*, 314-319.

O'Connor, G., and Drennan, C. (2003). Optimising patient care: meeting the needs of the paediatric oncology patient. *Journal of Diagnostic Radiography and Imaging, 5*, 33-38.

Pan, H., Chiu, P., Shen, J., and Chen, C. (2004). Application of therapeutic play in the process of nursing a preschool patient. *Journal of Nursing (China), 51*, 94-100.

Penkman, L., Scott-Lane, L., and Pelletier, W. (2006). A psychosocial program for pediatric oncology patients: A pilot study of "The Beaded Journey." *Journal of Psychosocial Oncology, 24*, 103-115.

Polit, D. F., and Beck, C. T. (2008). *Nursing research: Generating and assessing evidence for nursing practice* (8th ed.). Philadelphia: Lippincott Williams and Wilkins.

Radloff, L. S. (1977). A CES-D scale: A self-report depression scale for research in the general population. *Apply Psychology Measurement, 1*, 385-401.

Ribeiro, P. J., Sabates, A. L., and Riberio, C. A. (2001). The use of a therapeutic toy as an instrument of nursing intervention when preparing the child to blood collection. *Revista da Escola de Enfermagem da USP, 35*, 420-428.

Schultheis, M. T., and Rizzo, A. A. (2001). The application of virtual reality technology in rehabilitation. *Rehabilitation Psychology, 46*, 296-311.

Smallwood, S. B. (1988). Preparing children for surgery. *AORN Journal, 47* (1), 177-185.

Stam, H., Grootenhuis, M. A., Caron, H. N., and Last, B. F. (2006). Quality of life and current coping in young adult survivors of childhood cancer: Positive expectations about the further course of the disease were correlated with better quality of life. *Psycho-Oncology, 15*, 31-43.

Steele, E., Grimmer, K., Thomas, B., Mulley, B., Fulton, I., and Hoffman, H. (2003). Virtual reality as a pediatric pain modulation technique: A case study. *CyberPsychology and Behavior, 6,* 633-638.

Stewart, S. M., Lam, T. H., Betson, C., and Chung, S.F. (1999). Suicide ideation and its relationship to depressed mood in a community sample of adolescents in Hong Kong. *Suicide and Life-Threatening Behavior,* 29, 227-240.

Sung, L., Yanofsky, R., Klaassen, R. J., Dix, D., Pritchard, S., Winick, N., Alexander, S., Klassen, A. (2011). Quality of life during active treatment for pediatric acute lymphoblastic leukemia. *International Journal of Cancer, 128*, 1213-1220.

Vessey, J. A., and Mahon, M. M. (1990). Therapeutic play and the hospitalized child. *Journal of Pediatric Nursing, 5*(5), 328-333.

Weiss, P.L., Bialik, P., and Kizony, R. (2003). Virtual reality provides leisure time opportunities for individuals with physical and intellectual disabilities. *CyberPsychology and Behavior, 6*, 355-342.

Weissman, M. M., Orvaschel, H., and Padian, N. (1980). Children's symptom and social functioning self-report scales: comparison of mothers' and children's reports. *The Journal of Nervous and Mental Disease, 168,* 736-40.

Whitsett, S. F., Gudmundsdottir, M., Davies, B., McCarthy, P., Friedman, D. (2008). Chemotherapy-related fatigue in childhood cancer: correlates, consequences, and coping strategies. *Journal of Pediatric Oncology Nursing*, 25, 86-96.

Williams, P., Schmideskamp, J., Ridder, L., and Williams, A. (2006). Symptom monitoring and dependent care during chemotherapy in children. *Cancer Nursing, 29*(3), 188-197.

In: Pediatric Cancer
Editor: William Li

ISBN: 978-1-61942-112-7

Chapter 4

Understanding how Children Coped with Cancer: An Essential Prerequisite for Designing Appropriate Psycho-Educational Interventions

William H. C. Li
School of Nursing, Li Ka Shing Faculty of Medicine
The University of Hong Kong, Hong Kong S.A.R., China

Abstract

Notwithstanding the increasing survival rates for childhood cancers, the course of treatment for cancer, such as chemotherapy, surgery or radiotherapy, is still a very stressful experience in the life of a child and may lead to long term physical, emotional and psychosocial damage for children. There is some evidence that both chemotherapy and radiotherapy may have adverse effects upon normal body tissue that may manifest themselves months or even years after completion of the therapy. However, children with cancer may not only be at risk from adverse medical effects, their psycho-social well being, self-esteem and quality of life may also be severely affected as a result of their cancer and its therapy. There is an imperative need for nurses to develop and evaluate interventions that can help to ease the burden of cancer treatment for children. First, however, knowing how children coped with the diagnosis and treatment of cancer is a crucial step toward designing appropriate psycho-educational interventions.

A cross-sectional study was employed. Eighty-eight Hong Kong Chinese children aged 9 to 16 years, admitted for treatment of cancer in a paediatric oncology unit of an acute public hospital, were invited to participate in the study. To understand how children coped with their illness and responded to the diagnosis and treatment of cancer, they were asked to respond to the Coping Behaviour Checklist for Chinese Children on day 7 after admission or before discharge.

The results of this study revealed that Hong Kong Chinese children and their Western counterparts adopted different strategies for coping with cancer. The findings indicated that self-control (emotion-focused) was the most commonly reported coping strategy used by Hong Kong Chinese children. The results of this study is incongruent with previous studies on Western children in which it was found that seeking social support (problem-focused) was the most commonly reported coping strategy. On the other hand, this study revealed that children used different coping strategies at different developmental stages, with younger children (aged 9-12) used less problem-focused and more emotion-focused coping strategies than older children (aged 13-16).

An understanding of the coping behaviour of children is an essential prerequisite for the design of an appropriate psycho-educational intervention to reduce the children's emotional distress and bolster their coping mechanisms. This study has addressed a gap in the literature by examining how Hong Kong Chinese children coped with and responded to the diagnosis and treatment of cancer. It is anticipated that the information derived from this study can make a contribution to the advancement of nursing knowledge. Most importantly, the findings from this study can help nurses to shape and design appropriate psychological interventions that can help to reduce the burden of the cancer treatment and promote normal growth and development for children with cancer.

INTRODUCTION

Treatment of cancer constitutes a stressful and anxiety-provoking experience, which can be emotionally devastating for children. The course of treatment for cancer may incorporate chemotherapy, surgery, radiotherapy, and bone marrow transplantation, alone or in combination, all of which may severely affect children's physical well-being. In a study to examine the impact of cancer on children's physical well-being (Li, Chung, and Chiu, 2010), the results revealed that children most often viewed pain resulting from diagnostic procedures and medical treatments as one of the worst aspects of their cancer experience. Besides, nausea and vomiting, loss of appetite, feeling sluggish, stomatitis and fever were the most common treatment-related symptoms reported by children hospitalized with cancer. Langeveld, Grootenhuis, Voute, Hann, and Bos (2004) point out that both chemotherapy and radiotherapy may have adverse effects on normal body tissue, manifested moths or even years after the completion of treatment. For better control of cancer and prevent second malignancies, children with cancer are often required more than one treatments at a time (Children's Cancer Foundation, 2011). It is believed that children receiving combined treatment generally experienced greater severity of symptoms than those other children receiving single type of treatment. This is because, as every cancer treatment has unique and similar side effects on physiological well-being, and children receiving more than one treatment may well experience more, and more severe, treatment-related symptoms.

Cancer and its treatment may not adversely affect the physical well-being of children, but their psycho-social well being (Langeveld, et al., 2004). Previous studies indicate that irradiation, chemotherapy and surgical intervention may have long-term effects on the psychosocial well-being of children, including self-esteem, anxiety and depression, severely affecting their quality of life (Essen, Enskär, Kreuger, Larsson, and Sjödén, 2000; Li et al., 2010; Stam, Grootenhuis, Caron, and Last, 2006).

There are possible reasons that may explain why the psycho-social well-being of children with cancer can be adversely affected. First, children who had cancer as children are likely to have experienced many life-threatening traumas, invasive medical procedures and long periods of hospitalisation, and more recent health threats related to side effects or potential cancer recurrence (Schwartz and Drotar, 2006). Second, children are more vulnerable to the stress of illness than adults because of their limited cognitive capacities, lack of self-control and greater dependence on others (Li, Lopez, and Lee, 2007). Additionally, children's inability to understand the reasons for their illness and treatment can add to their anxiety, fear, anger, uncertainty and feelings of helplessness (Li, et al., 2007).

Given the issue of cancer and its treatment have tremendous impact on children's physical and psycho-social well-being, there is an imperative need for nurses to develop and evaluate interventions that can help to ease the burden of cancer treatment and its side effects for children. First, however, careful assessment the coping processes of children with cancer, especially the ways they think they will cope, is a necessary step towards designing appropriate interventions to promote their psychosocial well-being. The ways which children use to cope with and respond to the illness may differ, which is susceptible to cultural differences (Li, 2009). Lazarus and Folkman (1984) point out that differences in the ways in which individuals cope may be expected to affect each person's response to a psychological intervention. A comprehensive review of the mental health of children reveals that there are differences in the cognitive behaviour of Hong Kong Chinese children when compared with their Western counterparts (Wong and Tsoi, 1999). Hong Kong Chinese children are more submissive, and generally lack creativity, and creative thinking when compared with Western children. This may be the result of Hong Kong's socio-cultural emphasis on obedience and social conformity, academic performance, inhibition of self-expression, and avoidance of being deviant or making mistakes (Tsoi and Pryde, 1999). A recent longitudinal study to examine the relationships between perceived parental psychological control and psychological well-being in Hong Kong Chinese children revealed that parental psychological control may inhibit the development of positive mental well-being and affect emotional life in children (Shek, 2007). Conversely, it is well documented that Chinese culture is deeply influenced by the philosophical concepts of Confucianism (Chan, Cheung, Mok, Cheung, and Tong, 2006), and that this philosophy is reflected in certain notions of fatalism among Chinese people with respect to healthcare. They tend to believe that there is very little that can be done to change their fate, and therefore seem to think that life-threatening diseases such as cancer cannot be prevented (Li, 2009). Because the cultural context in which they live is drastically different from that of Western children, the way that Chinese children view the nature and meaning of their illness, as well as their responses to illness and psychosocial interventions, will also differ considerably from those of Western children.

The experience and coping behaviour of children with cancer have been researched in Western countries (Aldridge and Roesch, 2007; Dowling, Hockenberry, and Gregory, 2003; Whitsett, Gudmundsdottir, Davies, McCarthy, and Friedman, 2008).

Yet, a review of the literature reveals that, so far, very few studies have been conducted in the Hong Kong Chinese context. Given these issues, the study aimed to examine how Hong Kong Chinese children coped with cancer and its treatment. Specifically, what strategies that Hong Kong Chinese children used in coping with cancer were the focus.

Theoretical Framework

The present study was guided by Lazarus and Folkman's (1984) theory of cognitive appraisal, stress and coping, which is one of the most widely used theoretical perspectives examining how people cope with stress. This transactional model is also most frequently applied to research on children (Li *et al.* 2007; Su and Ryan-Wenger, 2007). However, like most such theories, Lazarus and Folkman's theory of coping is derived from the adult perspective. It has been recognised that the ways children cope are highly dependent on their psychosocial and cognitive development, which is distinctly different from that of adults (Peterson, 1989). In order to have a more thorough understanding of how children cope with stressful events, Piaget's (1963) theory of cognitive development, a developmental perspective, is also integrated into the framework of this study to provide essential complementary information on how children at different stages of development cope with a stressful situation.

According to Lazarus and Folkman (1984), coping is a process involving cognitive and behavioural attempts to meet the demands of a certain situation, and to control the emotions it generates. Lazarus and Folkman conceptualised coping as consisting of two categories: problem-focused and emotion-focused coping. Problem-focused coping is an activity aimed at modifying, avoiding or minimising the impact of the problem encountered, or an attempt to control the situation. Emotional-focused coping is based on the elimination of undesirable emotions that result from the stressful experience. Children may use either method of coping, or both, during the course of a stressful event. Lazarus and Folkman further categorised emotion-focused and problem-focused coping into eight coping strategies. Examples and definition of various coping strategies are shown in Table One. Problem-focused coping includes seeking social support, planned problem solving and confrontation. Emotion-focused coping includes positive reappraisal, self-control, escape avoidance, accepting responsibility and distancing. Lazarus and Folkman suggested that emotion-focused coping is the more common form used when nothing can be done to change the situation. Nevertheless, in order to manage the stress effectively in a specific situation, a person may use a variety of these coping strategies, individually or in combination.

Following the theoretical perspective of stress, appraisal and coping put forward by Lazarus and Folkman (1984), much research on how children cope with hospitalisation and medical procedures has been carried out (Dowling et al., 2003; LaMontagne, 2000; Ryan, 1989). LaMontagne (1984, 1987) examined the relationship between children's locus of control beliefs and their coping behaviour. The results of these studies provide some evidence that children with internal beliefs are more likely to adopt active coping behaviours (problem-focused coping), whereas children with an external orientation are more likely to adopt avoidance strategies (emotion-focused coping).

Piaget's theory provides a broad overview of cognitive development. According to Piaget (1963), children are born with a few sensorimotor schemata (elements in the organism's cognitive structure), which provide the framework for their initial interactions with the environment. The mechanisms that enable children to adapt to new situations and to move from one stage to the next are assimilation and accommodation.

Table 1. Examples and definition of emotion-focused and problem-focused coping strategies

Coping Strategy	Definition
Emotion Focused Coping	
Escape-Avoidance	Using wishful thinking and behavioural efforts to escape or avoid the stressful situation
Distancing	Creating a positive outlook by refusing to think too much or trying to forget about the stressful situation
Self-control	Making efforts to regulate one's own feelings or emotions
Accepting Responsibility	Acknowledging one's own role in the problem and trying to put things right
Positive Reappraisal	Focusing on the positive aspects of the situation and / or personal growth
Problem-focused Coping	
Planful Problem Solving	Using an analytic approach to solve or manage the problem
Seeking Social Support	Making efforts to seek informational, tangible and emotional support from others
Confronting	Making aggressive efforts to alter the situation or openly expressing emotions

Piaget believed that children were actively involved in the construction of knowledge, incorporating new information into already existing knowledge structures or schemata, through assimilation.

When there was a new situation too different or too complex to be integrated into existing structures, the schemata were modified or expanded through the process of accommodation. Piaget also found that certain mental abilities tended to appear at certain stages of development, and believed that cognitive development involved a series of four separate stages in a fixed order: sensorimotor, pre-operational, concrete operational, and formal operational.

Each successive stage is defined by the appearance of a qualitatively different level of thinking, resulting in an increasingly sophisticated form of knowledge that provides greater intellectual balance for responding to the environment.

METHODS

Study Design and Sample

To examine how children coped with cancer, a cross-sectional study was employed in one of the largest acute-care hospitals in Hong Kong with a well-established paediatric oncology unit. Hong Kong Chinese children admitted for treatment of cancer, meeting the inclusion criteria for the study, were invited to participate in the study.

The inclusion criteria were: (1) all children should be aged 9 to 16 years, (2) children should be able to speak Cantonese and read Chinese, and (3) children should have been diagnosed with cancer for at least two months and be currently undergoing active medical treatment. We excluded children with cognitive and learning problems identified from their medical records. It is understandable that younger children may well be more vulnerable to the stress of cancer and its treatment. However, younger children may have limited verbal and cognitive capacities in expressing themselves and be perplexed by the questionnaire.

In this connection, only children aged 9-16 years were invited to participate in the study. A total of 88 children hospitalized with cancer were recruited during an 8-month period from 2008 to 2009. The response rate was 98%, with only two sets of parents, without giving any specific reasons, choosing not to participate.

Measurements

Demographic Data Sheet

A demographic data sheet was used to document children's demographic and clinical characteristics, such as age, gender, diagnosis and types of treatment received. In addition, parents' education attainment was also documented, which can provide indirect information that reflects the socio-economic status of a family.

The Coping Behaviour Checklist for Chinese Children (CBC-CC)

The CBC-CC originally was designed and developed as a research tool for documenting children's way of coping when faced with a stressful situation (Li, Chung, Wong, and Ho, 2010). The CBC-CC was used here to identify the coping strategies used by Hong Kong Chinese children hospitalized with cancer. The CBC-CC was developed according to concepts drawn from Lazarus and Folkman's (1984) theory of cognitive appraisal, stress and coping, which is one of the most frequently used theoretical perspectives on how people cope with stress.

Based on this framework, the CBC-CC aims to document children's coping behaviour on two dimensions: problem-focus and emotion-focused coping. Under each coping dimension, the CBCC contain subscales to document different coping strategies used by children. The CBC-CC asks children to indicate the way in which they would cope when faced with a very stressful event.

The CBC-CC consists of 8 items. The children are asked to indicate the frequency of occurrence of the behaviour described by each item by placing an X in the box corresponding to the response option that seems to fit them best. For each item the response options '*Hardly ever*,' '*Sometimes*,' and '*Often*' are offered, which is scored from 0 to 2, with total possible scores ranging from 0 to 16, and scores of 0 to 5, 6 to 10 and 11 to 16 are interpreted as corresponding to emotion-focused, mixed-focused and problem-focused responses, respectively.

The psychometric properties of the CBC-CC have been empirically tested, showing high content validity, appropriate construct validity, and adequate internal consistency reliability and test-retest reliability. The results of confirmatory factor analysis have added further evidence of the construct validity of the construct validity of the CBC-CC.

Study Procedure

Study approval was obtained from hospital ethics committees. Written consent was obtained from the parents after they were told the purpose of the study. They were given the option to participate or refuse their child's involvement in the study. The children were also invited to put their names on a special children's assent form and told that their participation was voluntary and were assured of the confidentiality of the study. On admission to the oncology unit, demographic data of children and their parents were collected by research nurse using the demographic sheet. The demographic data of the participants are shown in Table 2.

On day 7 after admission or before discharge, children were then asked how to cope with cancer and its treatment using the CBC-CC. In Hong Kong Chinese context, it is the common practice for physicians to disclose the cancer diagnosis of the child to parents and facilitate information sharing among family members (Yin and Twinn, 2004). However, to ascertain that children were aware they had cancer, the research nurse asked them the reasons for the admission to hospital before asking them to respond to the CBC-CC.

Data Analysis

The Statistical Package for Social Sciences (SPSS: Version 18.0; SPSS Inc., Chicago, IL, USA) for Windows was used for data analysis. Descriptive statistics were used to calculate the mean, standard deviation, and range of the scores of the demographic data and CBC-CC.

The relationships among the scores of the CB-CC and the participants' demographic data were investigated using the Pearson product-moment correlation coefficient. Because of children's age-linked cognitive development, the ways of coping with stressful situations may be different in younger and older children.

According to Piaget (1963), children at the ages of 9-12 and 13-16 are at the development stage of concrete operational and formal operational stages, respectively. Therefore, the coping strategies used by children of different age groups were assessed by chi-square test.

Table 2. Demographic Characteristics of the Participants (*n* = 88)

Age (yrs)	Frequency	%
9	13	14.8 %
10	14	15.9 %
11	11	12.5 %
12	11	12.5 %
13	13	14.8 %
14	12	13.6%
15	8	9.1%
16	6	6.8%
Sex		
Male	47	53.4 %
Female	41	46.6 %
Diagnosis		
Leukemia	39	44.3 %
Lymphoma	26	29.5 %
Brain tumor	9	10.3 %
Germ-cell tumor	8	9.1 %
Osteoarcomas	6	6.8%
Types of treatment received		
Surgery	13	14.8 %
Chemotherapy	36	40.9 %
Bone Marrow Transplant	6	6.8 %
Mixed method	33	37.5 %
Education Attainment of parents		
Primary school or below	13	14.8 %
Lower secondary school	35	39.8 %
Upper secondary school	31	35.2 %
Tertiary education	9	10.2 %

RESULT

There were equal numbers of boys and girls, and most had been diagnosed with leukemia and lymphoma. Most participants (40.9%) received chemotherapy to treat their cancer, with 37.5% receiving more than one treatment. The overall results showed that 29.5% of children used problem-focused coping strategies, while 70.5% relied on emotion-focused coping. The interrelationships among the CBC-CC scores, age, sex, diagnosis, type of treatment received and education attainment of parents are shown in Table 3. With reference to Cohen (1992), correlation coefficients of 0.10 to 0.29, 0.30 to 0.49 and 0.50 to 1.0 are typically interpreted as small, medium, and large coefficients, respectively. The results showed that there was a high, positive correlation between CBC-CC scores and age.

Table 3. The intercorrelation coefficients among the CBC-CC scores, age, sex, diagnosis, type of treatment received, and education attainment of parents (N = 88)

A		B	C	D	E	F
Age (A)	1					
Sex (B)	0.52	1				
Diagnosis (C)	-0.09	0.06	1			
Type of treatment received (D)	-0.01	0.10	0.34a	1		
Education attainment of parents (E)	0.08	0.12	-0.16	-0.08	1	
CBC-CC (F)	0.58a	-0.06	-0.13	-0.11	0.21	1

Abbreviations: CBC-CC, the Coping Behaviour Checklist for Chinese Children.
[a] Significant at $p < 0.01$.

The coping strategies used by children of different age are shown in Table 4. A chi-square test revealed a statistically significant difference in coping strategies used between two age groups, with younger children (aged 9-12) used less problem-focused and more emotion-focused coping strategies than older children (aged 13-16).

DISCUSSION

Understanding how children cope with cancer is an essential prerequisite for designing appropriate psycho-educational interventions to ease the burden of cancer treatment. The aim of this study was to examine the coping strategies used by Hong Kong children hospitalized with cancer, an area of research that is under-represented in the existing literature.

The results showed that there was no statistically significant correlation among the CBC-CC scores, sex, diagnosis, types of treatment received and education attainment of parents. A review of the literature reveals that the results of previous studies on gender differences with respect to the use of coping strategies were found to be inconsistent. A longitudinal study of gender differences in the stressors and coping strategies of healthy school-aged children revealed that more girls than boys made use of social support and emotional expression (Sharrer and Ryan-Wanger, 1994).

Table 4. Coping strategies used by children of different age groups ($n = 88$)

	Age			
	9-12 (n = 48)	13-16 (n = 40)	χ^2	*p*
Coping strategies used	Frequency (%)			
Problem-focused Coping				
Seeking social support	11 (22.9)	6 (15.0)	20.35	0.005*
Planful problem solving	1 (2.1)	6 (15.0)		
Confronting	0 (0)	2 (5.0)		
Emotion-focused Coping				
Escape-avoidance	11 (22.9)	4 (10.0)		
Distancing	12 (25.0)	5 (12.5)		
Self-control	13 (27.1)	8 (20.0)		
Positive reappraisal	0 (0)	5 (12.5)		
Accepting responsibility	0 (0)	4 (10.0)		

* Significant at $p < 0.05$

These results were similar to those of another study that examined the ways children coped with chronic illness, in which more girls than boys used emotional regulation and social support (Spirito, Stark, Gril, and Tyc, 1995). This study also found that more boys than girls used cognitive restructuring (positive reappraisal) in coping with their chronic illness. Nevertheless, in accord with the present study, other research on children with acute or chronic illness has reported no significant gender differences in the coping strategies used (Bossert, 1994; Ryan-Wenger, 1994).

The result revealed that there was a high positive correlation between CBC-CC scores and age, with younger childhood cancer survivors (aged 9-12) using more emotion-focused and fewer problem-focused coping strategies than older survivors (aged 13-16). One possible reason for these differences is that the cognitive development of younger children is different from that of older children. The former have not yet achieved the cognitive maturity needed for a full understanding of the stressors encountered and for assimilating information. According to Piaget's (1963) theory of cognitive development, children in the 9-12 age group are all at the same developmental stage (concrete operational) in which they can develop logical reasoning about objects, events and relationships, but their thinking remains limited to concrete objects and events. They may not therefore have the cognitive ability to confront, re-appraise and accept responsibility when they encounter a stressful event. On the other hand, as children progress into the formal operational stage (12 years to adulthood), their thinking becomes logical and abstract and they can use a scientific approach to problem solving. Another possible reason is that as children become older, their locus of control shifts from an external to an internal focus (Li and Chung, 2009). Lefcourt (1982) believed that the increasing internality that evolves with age is probably due to the increased perception of control shaped by the individual's age or level of cognitive development. A previous study (LaMontagne, 1987) examined the relationship between locus of control beliefs of children and their coping behaviour found that children with a more externally focused locus of control are more likely to adopt emotion-focused coping strategies, whereas children with a more internally focused locus of control are more likely to adopt problem-focused strategies. This can explain why children use different coping strategies at different developmental stages.

The findings of the present study (Table 4) indicate that the most commonly reported coping strategy used by Hong Kong Chinese children is self-control (emotion-focused). In other words, many of them prefer to keep themselves calm and in control when faced with cancer. This finding is at odds with previous studies on Western children, where it was found that seeking social support (problem-focused) was the most commonly reported coping strategy (Aldridge and Roesch, 2007; Cole, Bruschi, and Tamang, 2002). In fact, the overall results of the present study reveal that Hong Kong Chinese children use more emotion-focused than problem-focused strategies. The findings are in accord with a previous study conducted among Hong Kong Chinese school children (Li et al., 2010) adding further evidence that Hong Kong Chinese people are influenced by the philosophy of Confucianism and the associated notion of fatalism. Under this influence, most Chinese childhood cancer survivors might believe that there was noting that could be done to change their situation. Lazarus and Folkman (1984) postulate that emotion-focused coping is the more common form used when nothing can be done to change the situation. This may explain why Hong Kong Chinese children use a more emotion-focused approach to cope with cancer.

Lazarus and Folkman (1984) categorized emotion-focused and problem-focused coping into eight strategies. However, Table 4 shows that only five coping strategies were identified in the age group 9-12, with two of which were problem-focused and three were emotion-focused. These results reveal that children in this age group would not use confronting, positive reappraisal and accepting responsibility as strategies to cope with cancer. This is understandable as the thinking processes of children are different from those of adolescents or adults. Younger children have not yet achieved the cognitive maturity needed for a full understanding of the stressors encountered and for assimilating information, and they have little experience of illness.

According to Piaget's (1963), children in the 7-12 age group can develop logical reasoning about objects, events and relationships, but their thinking remains limited to concrete objects and events. Younger children, such as the 9-12 age group of this study, may not therefore have the cognitive ability to confront, re-appraise and accept responsibility when they encounter a stressful event.

Piaget (1963) postulated that as children progress into the formal operational stage (12 years to adulthood), their thinking becomes logical and abstract and they can use a scientific approach to problem solving. Interestingly, the results of the present study reveal that only two children from the age group 13-16 used confronting as a strategy to cope with the treatment of cancer.

One possible explanation is that Chinese children in Hong Kong are influenced by the local socio-cultural emphasis on obedience and avoidance of being deviant or making mistakes (Tsoi and Pryde, 1999). They may therefore have learned to be more submissive, and thus to inhibit the expression of emotions such as hostility and anger when faced with a stressful event.

Implications for practice

Cancer and its treatment have tremendous impact on the physical and psychosocial well-being of children. Taking care of children with cancer therefore presents a major challenge to health care professionals. Indeed preparing children psychologically for invasive medical procedures, treatment and hospitalisation is one of the most vital responsibilities of a nurse.

The findings of the study have important implications for practice. First, this study highlights the importance of a careful assessment of children's coping behaviour, an essential prerequisite for the design of an effective and appropriate nursing intervention to enhance children's ability to cope with stressful medical procedures and hospitalisation. For example, as problem-focused coping is an activity aimed at modifying and minimizing the impact of the problem encountered, it is crucial for health care professionals to use interventions that include the provision of accurate information on details of sensory and procedural matters, allied to instructions which foster problem-solving activities. On the other hand, emotion-focused coping is based on the elimination of undesirable emotions that result from the stressful experience. It is therefore essential for health care professionals to develop interventions that attempt to regulate emotional distress by relaxation, distraction or denial to avoid any direct confrontation with the problem. Second, this study contributes to a better understanding of the ways of coping in Chinese children, an area of research that is under-represented in the existing literature. Third, through integrating Lazarus and Folkman's theory of coping and Piaget's theory of cognitive development into the theoretical framework of this study, it provides essential complementary information on how children at different developmental stages may use different coping strategies. Additionally, the findings of this study can be linked to Orem's (2001) general theory of nursing. This consists of three related theories: self care, self care deficit, and nursing system. According to the theory of nursing system, a nurse can assist a child to regulate self-care capabilities and meet therapeutic self-care requirements by providing appropriate nursing system (Foster and Bennett, 2002; Orem, 2001). The findings of this study can contribute to the development of supportive educative system, which is one of the nursing systems used to understand the patient's perspective on health and requirement of the self care system. These two components can be further influenced by the person's ways of coping. Therefore, it would be essential for a nurse to consider the ways of coping of children so as to help them to overcome the self-care deficits and ultimately enhance the quality of nursing care. Furthermore, the findings of this study can help shape the design of age-appropriate nursing interventions to promote children's coping with stressful medical procedures, treatments and hospitalization. Most importantly, the results of the study have the potential to increase nurses' knowledge and awareness of the impact of socio-cultural factors on children's coping. Indeed, there is an imperative need for nurses to be sensitive and knowledgeable about the cultural background of children before deciding how to prepare them to cope with stressful medical procedures.

Apart from contributing to the advancement of nursing knowledge, the findings of the study have some important implications for nursing practice. Owing to individual differences in coping can be expected to affect a person's response to psychological intervention, it is crucial for clinical nurses to assess carefully children's ways of coping according to their developmental stages on admission to hospital. Understanding the cognitive development and coping behaviour of children in advance can enhance the effectiveness of nursing intervention strategies in reducing anticipatory anxiety and bolstering their coping mechanisms during hospitalisation.

Limitation of the Study

Convenience sampling and the fact that all data were collected in one setting limits the ability to generalise the results. Besidess, due to small sample size was used in this study (88 participants), the findings might not produce sufficient evidence to state that there is difference in the ways of coping between Hong Kong Chinese children and their counterparts. More studies, particularly with larger samples, may be necessary to add more evidence on this issue. Another limitation is that only the most common coping strategy used by each child is identified, although Lazarus and Folkman suggested that, in order to manage the stress of a specific situation effectively, a variety of coping strategies can be used the person concerned, individually or in combination. Also, this study only compares the coping strategies used by children grouped according to sex, age group, diagnosis, types of treatment received and parents' educational attainment. However, other personal and situational factors, such as a child's locus of control and their previous experience with crises may well have an impact on the coping strategies used by the child. Therefore, a future study may consider using probability sampling to enhance the generalizability of the findings. In addition, further studies are needed to explore whether children would use either problem- or emotion-focused coping, or both, during the course of a stressful event. A future study should include more personal and situational factors in the data analysis so that a more thorough understanding the ways of coping of children can be achieved.

CONCLUSION

Despite its possible limitations, this study has addressed a gap in the literature by examining how Hong Kong Chinese children coped with cancer. It has found that Hong Kong Chinese children and their Western counterparts adopt different strategies for coping with cancer, and has also revealed that children use different coping strategies at different developmental stages. It is anticipated that the information derived from this study will help nurses design and shape appropriate psychological interventions that can help reduce the burden of cancer treatment and promote normal growth and development for children with cancer.

REFERENCES

Aldridge, A. A, and Roesch, S. C. (2007). Coping and adjustment in children with cancer: A meta-analytic study. *Journal of Behavior Medicine, 305*(2), 115-129.

Bossert, E. (1994). Factors influencing the coping of hospitalized school-age children. Journal of Pediatric Nursing, 9, 299-306.

Chan, E. A., Cheung, K., Mok, E., Cheung, S., and Tong, E. (2006). A narrative inquiry into the Hong Kong Chinese adults' concepts of health through their cultural stories. *International Journal of Nursing Studies,43*(3), 301-309.

Children's Cancer Foundation. Publications: Leaflets. Cancer in Children. http://www.ccf.org.hk/leaflet/all3.htm. Accessed May 22, 2010.

Cohen, J. (1992). A power primer. *Psychological Bulletin, 112*, 155-159.

Cole, P. M., Bruschi, C. J., and Tamang, B. L. (2002). Cultural differences in children's emotional reactions to difficult situations. *Child Development, 73*(3), 983-996.

Dowling, J. S., Hockenberry, M., and Gregory, R. L. (2003). Sense of humor, childhood cancer stressors, and outcomes of psychosocial adjustment, immune function, and infection. *Journal of Pediatric Oncology Nursing, 20*, 271-292.

Essen, L. V., Enskär, K., Kreuger, A., Larsson, B., and Sjödén, P. O. (2000) Self-esteem, depression and anxiety among Swedish children and adolescents on and off cancer treatment. *Acta Paediatrica,* 89, 229-236.

Foster, P. C., and Bennett, A. M. (2002). Self-care deficit nursing theory: D. E. Orem. In J. B. George (ed). *Nursing theories: The base for professional nursing practices*. New Jersey: Prentice Hall.

LaMontagne, L. L. (1984). Children's locus of control beliefs as predictors of preoperative coping behavior. *Nursing Research, 33*, 76-85.

LaMontagne, L. L. (1987). Children's preoperative coping: replication and extension. *Nursing Research, 36,* 163-167.

LaMontagne, L. L. (2000). Children's coping with surgery: A process-oriented perspective. *Journal of Pediatric Nursing, 5*, 307-312.

Langeveld, N. E., Grootenhuis, M. A., Voute, P. A., Haan, R. J., and Bos, C. V. D. (2004) Quality of life, self-esteem and worries in young adult survivors of childhood cancer. *Psycho-Oncology,* 13, 867-881.

Lazarus, R. S. (1984). Folkman S. *Stress, appraisal and coping*. New York: Springer.

Lefcourt HM. (1982). *Locus of control: Current trends in theory and research.* 2nd ed. Erlbaum, Hillsdale: NJ.

Li, H. C. W., Chung, O. K. J., Wong, E. M. L. and Ho, K. Y. E. (2010). Coping behaviour Checklist for Chinese children: development and psychometric testing. *Journal of Advanced Nursing,* 66(7), 1633-1643.

Li, H. C. W., Chung, O. K. J., and Chiu, S. Y. (2010). The impact of cancer on children's physical, emotional, and psychosocial well-being. *Cancer Nursing, 33*(1), 47-54.

Li, H. C. W., Lopez, V. and Lee, T. L. I. (2007). Effects of Preoperative Therapeutic Play on Outcomes of School-age Children Undergoing Day Surgery. *Research in Nursing and Health, 30,* 320-332.

Li, W. H. C. (2009). The Importance of Incorporating Cultural Issues into Nursing Interventions for Chinese Populations. In W.T. Chien (Eds). *Strategies in evaluation of complex health care interventions for people with physical or mental health issues*, New York: Nova Biomedical Book.

Li, W. H. C., and Chung, O. K. J. (2009). The relationship between children's locus of control and their anticipatory anxiety. *Public Health Nursing, 26*(2), 153-160.

Orem, D. E. (2001). Nursing concepts of practice (6th ed.). Mosby, St Louis, MO.

Peterson, L. (1989). Coping by children undergoing stressful medical procedures: Some conceptual, methodological and therapeutic issues. *Journal of Consulting and Clinical Psychology, 57*, 380-387.

Piaget, J. (1963) *The origins of intelligence in children*. New York: Norton.

Ryan, N. M. (1989). Stress-coping strategies identified from school age children's perspective. *Research in Nursing and Health, 12*, 111-122.

Ryan-Wenger, N. M. (1994). Coping behaviour in children: Methods of measurement for research and clinical practice. *Journal of Pediatric Nursing,* 9, 183-195.

Schwartz, L., and Drotar, D. (2006). Posttraumatic stress and related impairment in survivors of childhood cancer in early adulthood compared to healthy peers. *Journal of Pediatric Psychology, 31*(4), 356-366.

Sharrer, V., and Ryan-Wanger, N. (1994). A longitudinal study of age and gender differences of stressors and coping strategies in school-aged children. *Journal of Pediatric Health Care, 9*, 123-130.

Shek, D. T. L. (2007). A longitudinal study of perceived parental psychological control and psychological well-being in Chinese adolescents in Hong Kong. *Journal of Clinical Psychology, 63*(1), 1-22.

Spirito, A., Stark, L., Gril, K., and Tyc V. (1995). Coping with everyday and disease-related stressors by chronically ill children and adolescents. *Journal of the American Academy Child and Adolescent Psychiatry, 34*, 283-290.

Stam, H., Grootenhuis, M. A., Caron, H. N., and Last, B. F. (2006). Quality of life and current coping in young adult survivors of childhood cancer: Positive expectations about the further course of the disease were correlated with better quality of life. *Psycho-Oncology, 15*, 31-43.

Su, Y. H., and Ryan-Wenger, N. A. (2007). Children's adjustment to parental cancer: A theoretical model development. *Cancer Nursing, 30*(5), 362-381.

Tsoi, M. M., and Pryde, N. A. (1999). Hong Kong's children: overview and conclusion. In N. A. Pryde and M. M Tsoi (EDS.), *Hong Kong's Children: our past, their future* (pp. 573-647). Hong Kong: Centre of Asian Studies, the University of Hong Kong.

Whitsett, S. F., Gudmundsdottir, M., Davies, B., McCarthy, P., and Friedman, D. (2008). Chemotherapy-related fatigue in childhood cancer: correlates, consequences, and coping strategies. *Journal of Pediatric Oncology Nursing*, 25, 86-96.

Wong, C. K., and Tsoi, M. M. (1999). Mental health of Hong Kong Children. In N.A. Pryde and M.M. Tsoi (EDS.), *Hong Kong's Children: our past, their future* (pp. 153-220). Hong Kong: Centre of Asian Studies, the University of Hong Kong.

Yin, L. K., and Twinn, S. (2004). The effect of childhood cancer on Hong Kong Chinese families at different stages of the disease. *Cancer Nursing, 27*(1), 17-24.

In: Pediatric Cancer
Editor: William Li

ISBN: 978-1-61942-112-7

Chapter 5

THE PSYCHOSOCIAL WELL-BEING AND QUALITY OF LIFE OF CHILDHOOD CANCER SURVIVORS: AN EXPLORATORY STUDY

William H. C. Li
School of Nursing Studies, Li Ka Shing Faculty of Medicine
The University of Hong Kong, Hong Kong S.A.R., China

ABSTRACT

Recent advances in cancer screening and medical treatment for childhood cancer have dramatically improved survival rates. Yet, despite the improved prognosis, cancer survivors have to pay a high price in side effects, such as second malignancies, growth and endocrine dysfunction, and serious organ toxicities. Most of these health problems are considered late-emerging side effects of the chemotherapy and radiation treatments, which may manifest months or even years after the completion of treatment, severely affecting children's psychosocial well-being and quality of life. Whilst much of the effort has been paid to the physiological care of childhood cancer survivors, insufficient attention has focused on the impact of cancer and its treatment on the psychosocial well-being of childhood cancer survivors in Hong Kong. The aim of this study was to examine the impact of cancer on the psychosocial well-being and quality of life of Hong Kong Chinese childhood cancer survivors, an area of research that has been underrepresented in the literature.

To examine the impact of cancer on children, a cross-section study was employed. A total of 137 childhood cancer survivors, aged 9 to 16 years old, who had their medical follow-up at the out-patient clinic were invited to participate in the study. Participants were asked to respond to the Chinese version of the Centre for Epidemiologic Studies Depression Scale for Children, Rosenberg's Self-Esteem Scale and Pediatric Quality of Life Inventory. Additionally, a one-to-one qualitative interview was conducted with 10 participants randomly selected from the group.

The results of the study indicated that more than half of the participants were potentially at risk for depression, or at least presented some depressive symptoms. There were high negative correlations between depressive symptoms and self-esteem scores, and depressive symptoms scores and level of quality of life. Furthermore, a medium positive correlation was found between self-esteem scores and level of quality of life. The findings indicated that greater depressive symptoms reported by childhood cancer survivors were associated with lower self-esteem and poorer quality of life. Additionally, the study revealed that depressive symptoms are a strong predictor of quality of life of childhood cancer survivors.

The study reveals that cancer and its treatments have a tremendous impact on the psychosocial well-being and quality of life of survivors. It is essential for health care professionals to develop and evaluate appropriate interventions with the aims of promoting psychosocial well-being and enhancing the quality of life for these children. Most importantly, it is crucial to help them develop a positive view of the impact that the cancer experience has upon their life.

INTRODUCTION

Today's new technological and breakthroughs in the medical treatment of childhood cancer have dramatically improved survival rates than ever before (Li, Chung, and Chiu, 2010; Stam, Grootenhuis, Caron, and Last, 2006). According to the Hong Kong Cancer Registry (2009), the survival rates for most childhood cancers were close to 70%. Nevertheless, many studies reveal that cancer survivors have to pay a high price in side effects, such as second malignancies, growth and endocrine dysfunction, infertility, chronic hepatitis, impaired cognitive abilities, and serious organ toxicities (Hudson et al., 2003; Sharp, Kinahan, Didwania, and Stolley, 2007). Most of these chronic health problems are considered late-emerging side effects of the chemotherapy and radiation treatments. Langeveld, Grootenhuis, Voute, Haan, and Bos (2004) points out that both chemotherapy and radiotherapy may have adverse effects on normal body tissue, manifested months or even years after the completion of treatment.

Cancer and its treatments may not only adversely affect the physical well-being of childhood cancer survivors, but their psychosocial well-being as well (Langeveld et al., 2004). A review of the literature reveals that irradiation, chemotherapy and surgical intervention may have long-term effects on the psychosocial well-being of survivors, including self-esteem and depression (Essen, Enskär, Kreuger, Larsson, and Sjödén 2000; Stam et al., 2006; Zeltzer et al., 2009). Indeed, many previous studies conducted in Western countries reveal that such survivors are at high risk of depression (Michel, Rebholz, von der Weid, Bergstraesser, and Kuehni, 2010; Recklitis, Lockwood, Rothwell, and Diller, 2006). Moreover, in a childhood cancer survivor study, Schultz et al., (2007) reported that the children were 1.5 times more likely than their siblings to have symptoms of depression. Other studies have found that survivors report lower self-esteem and higher depression than healthy children (Essen et al., 2000; Servitzoglou, Papadatou, Tsiantis, and Vasilatou-Kosmidis, 2008). Additionally, there is some evidence that depressive symptoms predict suicidal tendencies (Ell, Sanchez, and Vourlekis, 2005; Stewart, Lam, Betson, and Chung, 1999). A large-scale surveillance in Hong Kong to examine the risk behaviours of school students revealed that around 25% of students with depressive symptoms had considered suicide and hurt themselves versus less than 10% amongst those without depressive symptoms (CUHK's School of Public Health, 2001).

The findings also revealed that those students with depressive symptoms were more likely to have unhealthy lifestyle, such as smoke, drink alcohol and take illicit drugs. In a study to examine the prevalence of suicidal ideation in survivors of childhood cancer, the results showed that the survivors are at an elevated risk for suicidal tendencies, even many years after treatment (Recklitis et al., 2006). The findings of these studies are alarming and warrant special attention by health care professionals.

There are certainly some reasons that may explain why the psychosocial well-being of these survivors can be adversely affected. First, survivors who had cancer as children are likely to have experienced many life-threatening traumas, invasive medical investigations and treatments, long periods of hospitalisation, and more recent health threats related to side effects or potential cancer recurrence (Schwartz and Drotar, 2006). Second, the physiological and psychological needs of children are significantly different from those of adults. Children are comparatively more vulnerable to the stress of illness and medical treatment than adults because of their limited cognitive capacities, lack of self-control, limited personal life experience and greater dependence on others. Additionally, children's failure to understand the reasons for their illness can add to their anxiety, fear, anger, uncertainty and feelings of helpness. Third, childhood cancer survivors may encounter new development tasks that are directly affected by the cancer and its side effects, which may then force them to revisit their cancer experience (Vannatta and Gerhardt, 2003).

Helping childhood cancer survivors maintain healthy psychosocial well-being, in particular enhancing their quality of life is one of the most vital responsibilities of a health care professional (Bradwell, 2009, Shepherd and Woodgate, 2010). Over the past decade, numerous Western studies have focused on developing and evaluating different psychosocial interventions for childhood cancer survivors (Andersen, Golden-Kreutz, Emery, and Debora, 2009; Hudson et al., 1998; Hudson, Tyc, Srivastava, Gattuso, Quargnenti, and Crom, 2002; Kazak, 2005). Interventions include psycho-educational, cognitive, behavioural and biological components have shown beneficial effects on psycho-social well-being of childhood cancer survivors. Yet, a review of the literature reveals that, so far, no similar study has been conducted in the Hong Kong Chinese context.

Whilst most local studies of childhood cancer have focused on examining the experience, psychological well-being and quality of life of family members or caregivers (Wills, 2009; Wong and Chan, 2006; Yiu and Twinn, 2001), the impact of cancer, in particular the side effects of treatment on the psychosocial well-being of survivors remain relatively underexplored. Although children with cancer in Hong Kong will receive regular medical follow-up after completing the entire course of treatment in a hospital, most attention has been focused on their physiological care. There is thus a compelling need for nurses in Hong Kong to provide long-term follow-up for survivors of childhood cancer, and to monitor the side effects of treatment on their psychosocial well-being.

Most importantly, it is crucial for nurses to develop and evaluate appropriate interventions that can promote the psychosocial well-being of such survivors and help them maintain a good quality of life. First, however, the impact of cancer and its treatments on the psychosocial well-being and quality of life of Hong Kong Chinese childhood survivors must be fully understood. Given these issues, the study aimed to examine the impact of cancer and its treatments on the psychosocial well-being and quality of life of Hong Kong Chinese childhood cancer survivors.

METHOD

Design

A cross-sectional study was employed. A total of 137 childhood cancer survivors in a paediatric oncology out-patient clinic were recruited during a 10-month period from 2010 to 2011.

Participants

Hong Kong Chinese childhood cancer survivors going through the medical follow-up procedures at the out-patient clinic of an acute-care hospital in Hong Kong and who met the study's inclusion criteria were invited to participate in the study. The definition of childhood cancer survivors here was children who had been diagnosed with cancer and were now at a minimum six-month stage after the completion of the entire course of hospital treatment.

The inclusion criteria were the following: (1) Hong Kong Chinese childhood cancer survivors; (2) all children should be aged 9 to 16 years; and (3) children should be able to speak Cantonese and read Chinese. We excluded children with evidence of recurrence or second malignancies, and those with cognitive and learning problems identified from their medical records. The response rate was 92% with 12 sets of parents choosing not to participate (without giving specific reasons).

Owing to the limited verbal and cognitive capacities of younger children in expressing themselves and they might be perplexed by the questionnaires, only children aged 9-16 years were invited to participate in the study.

According to Piaget (1963), children at the ages of 9-12 and 13-16 are at the development stage of concrete operational and formal operational stages, respectively. Piaget's (1963) claimed that children at the development stage of concrete operational can develop logical reasoning about objects, events and relationships, but their thinking remains limited to concrete objects and events.

They may not therefore have the cognitive ability to confront, re-appraise and accept responsibility when they encounter a stressful event. On the other hand, as children progress into the formal operational stage (12 years to adulthood), their thinking becomes logical and abstract and would be able to draw on more coping resources to deal with a stressful situation. The demographic data of the participants are shown in Table 1.

Table 1. Demographic Characteristics of the participants (N=137)

	Frequency	%
Age (yrs)		
9 - 12	71	51.9 %
13-16	66	48.1 %
Sex		
Male	70	51.1 %
Female	67	48.9 %
Diagnosis		
Leukemia	78	56.9 %
Lymphoma	30	21.9 %
Brain tumor	13	9.5 %
Osteoarcomas	10	7.3 %
Kidney tumor	4	2.9 %
Germ-cell tumor	2	1.5 %
Types of treatment received		
Surgery	5	3.6 %
Chemotherapy	66	48.2 %
Bone Marrow Transplant	6	4.4 %
Mixed method	60	43.8 %
Time since treatment was completed		
< 24 months	100	72.9 %
25 – 36 months	23	16.8 %
37 – 48 months	9	6.6 %
48 – 60 months	3	2.2 %
> 60 months	2	1.5 %
Education Attainment of parents		
Primary school or below	20	14.6 %
Lower secondary school	43	31.4 %
Upper secondary school	51	37.2 %
Tertiary education	23	16.8 %

Measurements

Demographic Data Sheet

A demographic data sheet was used to document children's demographic and clinical characteristics, such as age, gender, diagnosis, types of treatment received, and time since treatment was completed. In addition, parents' education attainment was also documented, which can provide indirect information that reflects the socio-economic status of a family.

The Center for Epidemiologic Studies Depression Scale for Children (CES-DC)

The CES-DC was derived from the Center for Epidemiologic Studies Depression Scale for Adult (CES-D) developed by Radloff (1977). The CES-D was then modified to become more child-friendly (Weissman, Orvaschel, and Padian, 1980). Additionally, the verbal attributes of the response scale were converted from absolute to relative categories. The CES-DC comprises 20 fully standardized items to evaluate depressive symptoms. The items consist of short and simple statements in the first person about the emotional, cognitive and behaviour related components of depressiveness. All items are evaluated on a four-point Likert scale in relation to their incidence during the last week, which were scored from 0 to 3 (0 = "not at all," 1 = "a lttle," 2 = "sometimes," 3 = "a lot"), with total possible scores ranging from 0 to 60, with higher scores indicating greater symptomatology. The cut-off point is fixed at 16. A score of 16 or greater indicates an individual demonstrating some depressive symptoms. The psychometric properties of the CES-DC have been empirically tested (Barkmann, Erhart, and Schulte-Markwort, 2008), showing adequate internal consistency reliability, good concurrent validity, and excellent construct validity. The results of confirmatory factor analysis showed that there are four factors underlying the CES-DC, which is congruent with hypothesized configuration of the factor structure of the CES-D proposed by Radloff (1977). The four-factor version of the CES-DC is considered to have good factorial validity and stability across age (Barkmann et al., 2008).

The psychometric properties of the Chinese version of the CES-DC have been empirically tested (Li, Chung, and Ho, 2010), showing adequate internal consistency reliability good content validity and appropriate convergent and discriminant validity. Confirmatory factor analysis added further evidence of the construct validity of the scale.

Rosenberg's Self-Esteem Scale (RSES)

The RSES was designed to measure self-esteem as a global disposition (Rosenberg 1965) and has been widely used with adolescents (Byrne, 2000; Kim, 2003) and children (Phillips, Bodfield, Woodthorpe, and Gimsley, 2008). The RSES consists of 10 items, an example being 'I am able to do things as well as most other people'. Responses are rated using a 4-point Likert scale ranging from 1 (strongly disagree) to 4 (strongly agree), with total possible scores ranging from 10 to 40. Higher scores indicate higher levels of self-esteem.

The Chinese version of the RSES has been used with adults (Chou and Chi, 2001; Ngai, Chan, and Eleanor, 2007), adolescents (Shek 2004, 2005) and children (Society for Community Organization, 2004). The results suggest that the Chinese version of the RSES can be used as a self-report assessment tool in measuring self-esteem of Chinese people.

Pediatric Quality of Life Inventory (PedsQL)

The PedsQL is a widely used scale to assess the health-related quality of life among children and adolescents between the age of 2 and 18 years (Varni, Burwinkle, Katz, Meeske, and Dickinson, 2002). It can be applied to both healthy children and paediatric patient population. The instrument consists of 23 items grouped into 4 subscales: physical functioning (8 items), emotional functioning (5 items), social functioning (5 items) and school functioning (5 items). Participants were asked how much of a problem has been experienced over the last month, which were scored from 0 to 4 (0 = never a problem, 1 = almost never a problem; 2= sometimes a problem, 3= often a problem, 4 = almost always a problem). The items are then reverse-scored and linearly transformed to a 0-100 scale (0 = 100, 1 = 75, 2 = 50, 3 = 25, 4 = 0). The scale scores were obtained by summing the items and dividing by the number of items of the scale. After transformation, scores range from 0 to 100, with higher scores indicating better health-related qualify of life.

The psychometric properties of the Chinese version of the PedsQL have been empirically tested (Chan, Chow, and Lo, 2005). Results suggest that the Chinese version of the PedsQL can be used as a reliable and valid measure of health-related quality of life in Chinese paediatric research and clinical application.

Semi-Structured Interview

To understand more thoroughly the impact of cancer and its treatment on the psychosocial well-being of childhood cancer survivors, in particular to find out what were the major concerns or worries that caused them to feel depressed or distress and consequently affected their quality of life, a one-to-one qualitative interview was conducted with 10 participants randomly selected from the group. Because of children's age-linked cognitive development, the impact of cancer and its treatment on psychosocial well-being may be different between younger and older children. Therefore, five childhood cancer survivors from each of the age group 9 to 12 and 13 to 16 were randomly selected for the qualitative interview.

The interviews were semi-structured and audio-taped. A detailed interview guide was used. Probing technique was used to elicit more comprehensive information. Repetition of original question and non-directive supplementary questions, such as "how is that?" or "why do you feel that way?" was asked for encouraging the children to give more detailed explanation regarding to their expressions.

Study Procedure

To ensure the rights of all participants were protected, especially for vulnerable subjects such as the children in this study, the researcher will strictly adhere to the Declaration of Helsinki (http://www.accreditgcp.com/download/Helsinki.pdf). This study was approved by the Institutional Review Board of the Hospital Authority Hong Kong West Cluster. Written consent was obtained from the parents after they were told the purpose of the study. They were given the option to participate or refuse their child's involvement in the study. The children were also invited to put their names on a special children's assent form and told that their participation was voluntary.

Childhood cancer survivors who underwent medical follow-up in the out-patient clinic were invited to participate in the study. After collection of the demographic data, all participants were asked to respond to the Chinese version of the CES-DC, the RSES, and the PedsQL.

After collection of quantitative data for all participants, 10 from the group were randomly selected for a semi-structured interview, which was conducted at their home. Each interview lasted approximately 30-45 minutes. To ensure the dependability and credibility of the data, some strategies were used in this study. First, to ensure the consistency in the conduct of interviews, one research nurse conducted all the interviews. The research nurse held the bachelor's degree in nursing and had experience in working with pediatric patients. Before commencing the interview, the research nurse received some training in communication skills with children by the researchers. She was asked to consider pace and intonation, simplicity, clarity and brevity, timing and relevance when choosing words to communicate with children. Second, to ensure the accuracy of the data by avoiding selective filtering of data through the researcher's recall and bias, all interviews were taped-recorded. Furthermore, to facilitate accurate interpretation of the data, field notes were recorded during and after interviews. Because the validity of data may be affected by children's eagerness to please their parents, causing them to respond the way they think their parents want them to respond, parents were encouraged not to stay with their child during the interview.

Data Analysis

The Statistical Package for Social Science (SPSS: Version 18; SPSS Inc., Chicago, IL, USA) for Windows was used for data analysis. Descriptive statistics were used to calculate the mean, standard deviation, and range of the scores of the different scales. The interrelationships among the scores of the different scales and demographic variables were investigated using the Pearson product-moment correlation coefficient. Because of children's age-linked cognitive development, the mean scores of the different scales of these the two age groups (9 to 12 and 13 to 16) were assessed by independent *t*-test. Multiple regression analysis was employed to explore whether depressive symptom and self-esteem could predict the quality of life of childhood cancer survivors while controlling for the possible effect of age, gender, diagnosis, type of treatment received, time since treatment was completed and education attainment of parents.

The study used content analysis and consensus coding in identification and categorization of reported physical and psychosocial well-being by the informants. After the interviews, the recording tape was immediately transcribed in Chinese and then translated into English by the research nurse. Transcription is a process that converts oral conversation into written form with dependability and credibility. Categories were identified by using data reduction approach. Two researchers carefully conceptualized the categories according to the similarities of the dialogues. Subsequently, all the transcribed interviews were sorted into different categories until each category was saturated. The concepts were then emerged by grouping similar categories together, and were named as codes.

After transcription coding, two researchers reviewed the codes. Differences in coding primarily arose from slight variations in the wording of statements. For further verification, peer debriefing was carried out. Peer debriefing involves sessions with peers to review different aspects of the inquiry. In this study, two nurse educators working in university with experience in data analysis of structured interview were consulted to review the codes and examine meaning until consensus was reached.

RESULT

The results showed that there were equal numbers of boys (51.1%) and girls (48.9%) and most of them had been diagnosed with leukemia (56.9%) and lymphoma (21.9%). More than half (72.9%) had completed the entire medical treatment within two years, with only two going on for more than five years. Results revealed that 52.6% of the participants were at or above the cut-off score of 16, indicating that, at least, they present some depressive symptoms.

The interrelationships among variables of CES-DC, RSES, PedsQL, and demographic variables are shown in Table 2. With reference to Cohen (1992), correlation coefficients of 0.10 to 0.29, 0.30 to 0.49 and 0.50 to 1.0 are typically interpreted as small, medium, and large coefficients, respectively. The results showed that there were high negative correlations between CES-DC and RSES scores, and CES-DC and PedsQL scores. Furthermore, a medium positive correlation was found between RSES and PedsQL scores.

The mean scores on the CES-DC, RSES, and PedsQL of the two age groups are shown in Table 3. An independent *t*-test showed that there was no statistically significant difference in mean CES-DC, RSES, and PedsQL scores between two age groups.

A summary of multiple regression analysis for variables (self-esteem and depressive symptoms) predicting quality of life of childhood cancer survivors is presented in Table 4. The results show that when all the variables are entered into the equation there are two variables (self-esteem and depressive symptom) that make a statistically significant contribution to predicting quality of life of childhood cancer survivors.

Based on content analysis and consensus coding in identification and categorization, four categories - physical, psychological, social and school dimensions - were identified.

Table 2. The intercorrelation coefficients among the CES-DC scores, CSAS-C scores, RSES scores, CBC-CC scores, PedsQL scores, age, sex, diagnosis, type of treatment received, time finished medical treatment and education attainment of parents (N = 137)

	A	B	C	D	E	F	G	H	I
Age (A)	1	0.52	-0.09	-0.01	0.43[a]	0.08	0.11	0.11	0.16
Sex (B)	0.52	1	0.06	0.10	-0.07	0.12	-0.07	0.12	0.06
Diagnosis (C)	-0.09	0.06	1	0.34[a]	-0.05	-0.16	0.11	-0.12	-0.16
Type of treatment received (D)	-0.01	0.10	0.34[a]	1	0.09	-0.08	-0.01	-0.08	0.01
Time since treatment was completed (E)	0.43[a]	-0.07	-0.05	0.09	1	0.12	-0.16	0.10	0.08
Education attainment of parents (F)	0.08	0.12	-0.16	-0.08	0.12	1	-0.04	0.06	0.13
CES-DC (G)	-0.11	-0.07	0.11	-0.01	-0.16	-0.04	1	-0.56[a]	-0.59
RSES (H)	0.11	0.12	-0.12	-0.08	0.10	0.06	-0.56[a]	1	0.43[a]
PedsQL (I)	0.16	0.06	-0.16	0.01	0.08	0.13	-0.59[a]	0.43[a]	1

Abbreviations: CES-DC, the Center for Epidemiologic Studies Depression Scale for Children; RSES, the Rosenberg's Self-Esteem Scale; PedsQL, Pediatric Quality of Life Inventory.

[a] Significant at $p < .01$.

Table 3. Mean scores for the CES-DC, CSAS-C, RSES, CBC-CC, PedsQL as listed by age groups

	Age			
	9 – 12 (n = 71)	13 -16 (n = 66)		
	Mean (SD)	Mean (SD)	t^a	p
CES-DC	16.92 (7.97)	15.83 (7.88)	0.79	.43
RSES	24.99 (4.92)	26.56 (5.85)	-1.71	.09
PedsQL	65.14 (16.97)	70.08 (14.39)	-1.83	.07

Abbreviations: CES-DC, the Center for Epidemiologic Studies Depression Scale for Children.

RSES, the Rosenberg's Self-Esteem Scale; PedsQL, Pediatric Quality of Life Inventory.

[a] Independent t-test.

Table 4. Summary of multiple regression for variables (therapy-related and depressive symptoms) predicting quality of life (N = 137)

Variable predicting quality of life	*B*	*SE B*	*β*	*p-value*
Step 1				
Age	0.58	0.55	0.13	0.29
Gender	2.10	1.81	0.10	0.25
Diagnosis	– 0.17	0.81	– 0.02	0.83
Type of treatment received	– 0.24	0.64	– 0.03	0.71
Time since treatment was completed	0.16	1.01	0.02	0.88
Education attainment of parents	0.44	0.98	0.04	0.65
Step 2				
Age	0.19	0.44	0.04	0.66
Gender	1.50	1.46	0.07	0.31
Diagnosis	0.60	0.65	0.07	0.37
Type of treatment received	0.23	0.51	0.03	0.65
Time since treatment was completed	0.62	0.88	0.07	0.48
Education attainment of parents	– 0.30	0.79	– 0.03	0.70
Depressive symptoms	– 0.68	0.11	– 0.52	<0.01
Self-esteem,	0.31	0.16	0.16	0.05
$R^2 = 0.39$				
Adjust $R^2 = 0.36$				
R^2 change = 0.36				

B = unstandardized coefficient; β = standardized coefficient; SE B = standard error of unstandardized coefficient.

DISCUSSION

Research indicates that increased survival rates are accompanied by an increase in associated physical and psychosocial problems. Whilst much of the attention has focused on the physiological care of childhood cancer survivors, the consequences of cancer and its treatments on psychosocial well-being and quality of life remain relatively underexplored. The aim of this study was to examine the impact of cancer on the psychosocial well-being and quality of life of Hong Kong Chinese childhood cancer survivors, an area of research that has been underrepresented in the literature.

The results of this study revealed that more than half of the participants were potentially at risk of depression, or at least presented some depressive symptoms as measured by the CES-DC. In comparison with previous studies (Li, Chan, Chung, and Chui, 2010; Li et al., 2010) using the same scale to measure depressive symptoms and self-esteem of a similar age group of Hong

Kong Chinese school children without cancer, the results revealed that the mean depressive symptom scores of childhood cancer survivor were relatively higher than those of school children without cancer, while the mean self-esteem scores of the survivor group were lower. The findings are consistent with previous studies from the West (Essen et al., 2000; Servitzoglou et al., 2008), showing that childhood cancer survivors report greater symptomatology of depression and lower self-esteem than healthy children. The results of this study also indicated that there were high correlations between CES-DC and RSES scores and CES-DC and PedsQL scores Again in accord with previous studies (Essen et al., 2000; Stam et al., 2006; Zeltzer et al., 2009), the present study indicates that greater symptomatology of depression in childhood cancer survivors is associated with lower self-esteem and poorer quality of life.

In childhood cancer survivors, feelings of depression may drag down self-esteem and even bring a higher risk of suicidal tendencies (Recklitis et al., 2006). Although it cannot be assumed from this cross-sectional study that there is a high risk of depression among childhood cancer survivors, many previous studies conducted in Western countries have revealed that childhood cancer survivors are at high risk of depression (Michel et al., 2010; Recklitis et al., 2006; Recklitis, Diller, Najita, Robison, and Zeltzer, 2010). For these reasons, the presentation of depressive symptoms in such survivors cannot be overlooked or underestimated. It is essential for healthcare professionals to detect and identify childhood cancer survivors with depressive symptoms at an early point, and subsequently take appropriate interventional steps to promote their psychosocial well-being.

On the other hand, there is some evidence that childhood depression may be caused by a negative psychological trait, such as low self-esteem (Cheung, 1996; Rosenberg, 1965). This study showed that self-esteem in childhood cancer survivors was associated with depression, anxiety and quality of life. Therefore, helping childhood cancer survivors to develop positive self-esteem can be a way to promote their psychosocial being and empower them to lead a healthier life.

In a previous study to examine the relationships among therapy-related symptoms, depressive symptoms and quality of life in Chinese children hospitalized with cancer (Li, Williams, Lopez, Chung, and Chiu, in press), the results indicated that children receiving combined cancer treatment generally experienced greater severity of symptoms and children reporting greater symptom severity experienced higher levels of depression and a lower level of quality of life. Furthermore, a medium positive correlation between type of treatment received and depressive symptoms scores and a medium negative correlation between type of treatment received and quality of life were found. The results of present study show that there was no statistically significant correlation among the variables of the CES-DC, RSES and PedsQL and the participants' demographic data, including type of treatment received. One possible reason is that participants in this study were at least at a minimum six-month stage after the completion of the entire course of treatment, which has no longer effects on their psychosocial well-being and quality of life. Nevertheless, the finding is at odds with the Western literature, where it is reported that variables including cancer diagnosis, type of treatment received, age, socio-economic factors and number of years since treatment completed might have different effects on the experience of childhood cancer survivors.

A multiple regression analysis was performed to examine whether self-esteem and depressive symptoms can predict the quality of life of childhood cancer survivors, after controlling for the possible effects of age, gender, diagnosis, type of treatment received, time since treatment was completed and parents' education attainment. The result showed that the overall model explained 39% of the variance. After controlling for the possible effects of age, gender, diagnosis and type of treatment, it was found that the R^2 change value was 0.36 - that is, self-esteem and depressive symptoms explained an additional 36% of the variance in quality of life. With all variables entered into the equation, there were two – self-esteem and depressive symptoms – that made a statistically significant contribution ($p < 0.05$), implying that these two factors could predict the quality of life of childhood cancer survivors. However, beta coefficients for type of treatment received, self-esteem and depressive symptoms were 0.16, –0.52 respectively, indicating that depressive symptoms formed a comparatively strong predictor of quality of life of childhood cancer survivors.

To explore further the impact of cancer and its treatment on the physical and psychosocial well-being of childhood cancer survivors, qualitative interviews were conducted to 10 participants randomly selected from the group. They were asked about their experience of cancer, in particular how the disease and its treatment had affected their daily life. In respect of the impact of cancer on physical well-being, most of the children reported that fatigue, memory loss, poor concentration and activity intolerance were their major concerns, many informants saying they easily felt tired even with adequate rest. The most annoying issue related to a decreased attention span, which caused them learning difficulties at school and when studying at home.

As for the psychological dimension, the issues most frequently talked about by children in the interviews were uncertainty and fear. As there is no 100% guarantee that the cancer will not come back, cancer recurrence and second malignancies became a constant fear for the survivors. In the social dimension, owing to the decrease in physical strength and endurance after remission, some children complained that they could no longer participate in some games as before. Additionally, because of their relatively low body resistance and high susceptibility to infection, many parents did not allow them near crowded public places, in particular during the seasonal outbreak of influenza, consequently affecting their normal social life and weakening social bonds. One of the rare positive effects that the cancer experience had on their lives, however, was the enhancement of their family relationships. Most childhood cancer survivors reported that they gained more psychological support and encouragement from their parents and siblings, which made them feel they were not alone. Lastly, as far as school was concerned, many informants reported that they were anxious about their academic performance, which they claimed was significantly affected by the cancer and its treatment. The cultural context in Hong Kong is one where Chinese parents place a considerable emphasis on academic performance and they regard academic achievements as the top priority in child care (Li and Chung, 2009). Given this cultural context, Hong Kong Chinese children are under tremendous pressure to excel in academic performance. Indeed, as a result of suspension from school during the course of treatment, a decreased attention span and excessive tiredness after remission, they had to make extra efforts to catch up with their studies.

Implications for Practice

Childhood cancer survivors are at risk of adverse physical and psychosocial effects of the cancer treatment, resulting from chemotherapy toxicities, radiation or secondary cancers. The side effects may even last many years after completion of treatment, severely affecting children's psychosocial well-being and quality of life. Nevertheless, insufficient attention has been paid to the impact of cancer and its treatment on the psychosocial well-being of childhood cancer survivors in Hong Kong. This study revealed that a significant number of such survivors in Hong Kong suffered from low self-esteem and experienced high levels of depression. Indeed, ensuring physical and psychosocial well-being in childhood cancer survivors should be a prime concern of healthcare professionals. It is crucial to develop and evaluate interventions that can help these children to engage in healthy lifestyles, and to provide psychosocial support at every step of their long and difficult journey.

Apart from contributing to the understanding of the impact of cancer and its treatments on childhood cancer survivors, the findings have important implications for practice. As self-esteem is moderately stable over time, it can be a useful indicator for screening those children who are likely to exhibit psychosocial distress or are at high risk of depression. Understanding the self-esteem of childhood cancer survivors in advance could therefore increase the effectiveness of interventions to help them develop positive self-esteem, thus promoting their psychosocial well-being.

On the other hand, the study revealed that depressive symptoms are a strong predictor of quality of life of childhood cancer survivors. It is crucial therefore for nurses to be sensitive and knowledgeable about the depressive symptoms of childhood cancer survivors and its effects on children's quality of life. Most importantly, there is an imperative need for nurses to detect and identify childhood cancer survivors with depressive symptoms at an early point. Early identification of depressive symptoms in childhood cancer survivors could help nurses to develop appropriate and effective interventions with the aims of alleviating their depressive symptom severity, and thus promoting the child's psychosocial well-being and quality of life.

Study limitations

The use of convenience sampling and all data were collected in one setting mean that the extent to which the results of this study can be generalized is limited. Additionally, we did not obtain information from parents on the psychosocial well-being of their children, which might have further enhanced our understanding of the impact of childhood cancer and its treatments on the survivors.

Conclusion

Despite its possible limitations, this study has addressed a gap in the literature by examining the impact of cancer and its treatments on the psychosocial well-being, in particular the depressive symptoms, self-esteem and quality of life of Hong Kong Chinese childhood cancer survivors. The study reveals that cancer and its treatments have a tremendous impact on the psychosocial well-being and quality of life of survivors. It is essential for health care professionals to develop and evaluate appropriate interventions with the aims of promoting psychosocial well-being and enhancing the quality of life for these children. Most importantly, it is crucial to help them develop a positive view of the impact that the cancer experience has upon their life.

REFERENCES

Andersen, B. L., Golden-Kreutz, D. M., Emery, C. F., and Debora, L. T. (2009) Biobehavioral Intervention for Cancer Stress: Conceptualization, Components, and Intervention Strategies. *Cognitive and Behavioral Practice,* 16(3), 253-265.

Barkmann, C., Erhart, M., and Schulte-Markwort, M. (2008). The German version of the Centre for Epidemiological Studies Depression Scale for Children: psychometric evaluation in a population-based survey of 7 to 17 years old children and adolescents – results of the BELLA study. *European Child and Adolescent Psychiatry,* 17, 116-124.

Bradwell, M. (2009). Survivors of childhood cancer. *Pediatric Nursing* 21(4), 21-24.

Byrne, B. (2000). Relationship between anxiety, fear, self-esteem and coping strategies in adolescence. *Adolescence,* 35(137), 215-301.

Chan, L. F. P., Chow, S. M. K, and Lo, S. K. (2005). Preliminary validation of the Chinese version of the pediatric quality of life inventory. *International Journal of Rehabilitation Research*, 28(3), 219-227.

Cheung, S. K. (1996). Reliability and factor structure of the Chinese version of the Depression Self-rating Scale. *Education and Psychological Measurement*, 56(1), 142-154.

Chou, K. L., and Chi, I. (2001) Social comparison in Chinese older adults. *Aging and Mental Health,* 5(3), 242-252.

Cohen, J. (1992). A power primer. *Psychological Bulletin, 112*, 155-159.

CUHK's School of Public Health. (2001). *New health crisis of our young generation: Surveillance finds many school students are emotionally disturbed.* http://www.breakthrough.org.hk/ir/youthdatabank/index.htm (accessed 20 May 2011).

Ell, k., Sanchez, K., and Vourlekis, B. (2005) Depression, receipt of depression care, and correlates of depression among low-income women with breast or gynecological cancer. *Journal of Clinical Oncology*, 23, 3052-3060.

Essen, L. V., Enskär, K., Kreuger, A., Larsson, B., and Sjödén, P. O. (2000). Self-esteem, depression and anxiety among Swedish children and adolescents on and off cancer treatment. *Acta Paediatrica,* 89, 229-236.

Hong Kong Cancer Registry, Hospital Authority (2009). Hong Kong Cancer Stat 2007. http://www3.ha.org.hk/cancereg/e_canstat2007.pdf. Accessed May 18, 2011.

Hudson, M. M., Hinds, P. S., Tyc, V., Gattuso, J., Quargnenti, A., Srivastava, D. K., Crom, D. B. and Mason, C. (1998). An educational intervention to improve health knowledge and behavior in childhood cancer survivors. *Journal of Pediatric Oncology Nursing*, 15(2), 112-113.

Hudson, M. M., Mertens, A. C., Yasui, Y., Hobbie, W., Chen, H., Gurney, J. G., Yeazel, M., Reckitis, C. J., Marina, N., Robison, L. R., and Oeffinger K.C. (2003). Health status of adult long-term survivors of childhood cancer: A report from the Childhood Cancer Survivor Study. *Journal of the American Medical Association,* 290, 1583-339.

Hudson, M. M., Tyc, V. L., Srivastava, D. K., Gattuso, J., Quargnenti, A. and Crom, D. B. (2002). Multi-component behavioral intervention to promote health protective behaviors in childhood cancer survivors: the protect study. *Medical and Pediatric Oncology,* 39, 2-11.

Kazak, A. E. (2005). Evidence-based interventions for survivors of childhood cancer and their families. *Journal of Pediatric Psychology,* 30(1), 29-39.

Kim, Y. H. (2003). Correlation of mental health problems with psychological constructs in adolescence: final results from a 2-year study. *International Journal of Nursing Studies,* 40, 115-124.

Langeveld, N. E., Grootenhuis, M. A., Voute, P. A., Haan, R. J., and Bos, C. V. D. (2004). Quality of life, self-esteem and worries in young adult survivors of childhood cancer. *Psycho-Oncology, 13*, 867-881.

Li, H. C. W., Chung O. K. J. and Chiu, S. Y. (2010). The impact of cancer on children's physical, emotional, and psychosocial well-being. *Cancer Nursing,* 33(1), 47-54.

Li, H. C. W., Chung, O. K. J. and Ho, K. Y. E. (2010) Psychometric Testing of the Chinese version of the Center for Epidemiologic Studies Depression Scale for Children. *Journal of Advanced Nursing, 66(11), 2582-2591.*

Li, W. H. C., Chan, S. L. P., Chung, O. K. J. and Chui, M. L. M. (2010) Relationships among mental health, self-esteem and physical health in Chinese adolescents: an exploratory study. *Journal of Health Psychology,* 15(1), 96-106.

Li, W. H. C., Chung, O. K. J. (2009). The relationship between children's locus of control and their anticipatory anxiety. *Public Health Nursing,* 26(2), 153-160.

Li, H. C. W., Williams, P. D., Lopez, V., Chung, J. O. K., and Chiu, S. Y. (in press). Relationships among therapy-related symptoms, depressive symptoms and quality of life in Chinese children hospitalized with cancer: An exploratory study. *Cance Nursing.*

Michel, G., Rebholz, C. E., von der Weid, N. X., Bergstraesser, E., and Kuehni, C. E. (2010). Psychological distress in adult survivors of childhood cancer: the Swiss Childhood Cancer Survivor study. *Journal of Clinical Oncology,* 28(10), 1740-1748.

Ngai, F. W., Chan, W. C. S., and Eleanor, H. (2007). Translation and validation of a Chinese version of the Parenting Sense of Competence Scale in Chinese monthers. *Nursing Research, 56,* 348-354.

Phillips, D., Bodfield, E., Woodthorpe, K., and Gimsley, M. (2008). Exploring the impact of group work and mentoring for multiple heritage children's self-esteem, well-being and behaviour. *Health and Social Care in the Community,* 16(3), 310-321.

Piaget, J. (1963). *The origins of intelligence in children.* New York: Norton.

Radloff, L. S. (1977). A CES-D scale: A self-report depression scale for research in the general population. *Applied Psychological Measurement,* 1, 385-401.

Recklitis, C. J., Diller, L. R., Najita, J., Robison, L. L., and Zeltzer, L. (2010). Suicide ideation in adult survivors of childhood cancer: a report from the Childhood Cancer Survivor Study. *Journal of Clinical Oncology,* 28(4), 655-661.

Recklitis, C. J., Lockwood, R. A., Rothwell, M. A., and Diller, L. R. (2006). Suicidal ideation and attempts in adult survivors of childhood cancer. *Journal of Clinical Oncology,* 24(24), 3852-3857.

Rosenberg, M. (1965). *Society and Adolescent Self-image.* Princeton University Press, Princeton.

Schultz, K. A. P., Ness, K. K., Whitton, J., Recklitis, C., Zebrack, B., Robison, Zeltzer, L., and Mertens, A. C. (2007). Behavioural and social outcomes in adolescent survivors of childhood cancer: A report from the childhood cancer survivor study. *Journal of Clinical Oncology, 25*(24), 3649-3656.

Schwartz, L., and Drotar, D. (2006). Posttraumatic stress and related impairment in survivors of childhood cancer in early adulthood compared to healthy peers. *Journal of Pediatric Psychology, 31*(4), 356-366.

Servitzoglou, M., Papadatou, D., Tsiantis, I., and Vasilatou-Kosmidis, H. (2008). Psychosocial functioning of young adolescent and adult survivors of childhood cancer. *Support Care Cancer Support Care Cancer,* 16, 29-36.

Sharp, L. K., Kinahan, K. E., Didwania, A., and Stolley, M. (2007). Quality of life in adult survivors of childhood cancer. *Journal of Pediatric Oncology Nursing,* 24(4), 220-226.

Shek, D. T. L. (2004). Chinese cultural beliefs about adversity: Its relationship to psychological well-being, school adjustment and problem behavior in Chinese adolescents with and without economic disadvantage. *Childhood, 11*, 63-80.

Shek, D. T. L. (2005). Paternal and maternal influences on the psychological well-being, substance abuse, and delinquency of Chinese adolescents experiencing economic disadvantage. *Journal of Clinical Psychology, 61*, 219-234.

Shepherd, E. J. W., and Woodgate, R. L. (2010). Cancer Survivorship in children and young adults: A concept analysis. *Journal of Pediatric Oncology Nursing,* 27(2), 109-118.

Society for Community Organization. (2004). Today's Children. Future of Hong Kong: A survey report. Society for Community Organization.

Stam, H., Grootenhuis, M.A., Caron, H. N., and Last, B. F. (2006) Quality of life and current coping in young adult survivors of childhood cancer: Positive expectations about the further course of the disease were correlated with better quality of life. *Psycho-Oncology,* 15, 31-43.

Stewart, S. M., Lam, T. H., Betson, C., and Chung, S.F. (1999). Suicide ideation and its relationship to depressed mood in a community sample of adolescents in Hong Kong. *Suicide and Life-Threatening Behavior,* 29, 227-240.

Vannatta, K., and Gerhardt, C. A. (2003). Pediatric oncology: Psychosocial outcomes for children and families. In M. C. Roberts (Ed.), *Handbook of Pediatric Psychology* (3rd ed., pp. 324-357). New York: Guilford Press.

Varni, J. W., Burwinkle, T. M., Katz, E. R., Meeske, K., and Dickinson, P. (2002). The PedsQL™ in pediatric cancer: Reliability and validity of the pediatric quality of life inventory™ generic core scale, multidimensional fatigue scale and cancer module. *Cancer, 94*(7), 2090-2106.

Weissman, M. M., Orvaschel, H., and Padian, N. (1980). Children's Symptom and Social Functioning Self-report Scales comparison of mothers' and children's reports. *The Journal of Nervous and Mental Disease,* 168(12), 736-740.

Wills, B. S. H. (2009). Coping with a child with acute lymphocytic leukemia. *Cancer Nursing,* 32(2), E8-E14.

Wong, Y. F. M., and Chan, W. C. S. (2006). The qualitative experience of Chinese parents with children diagnosed of cancer. *Journal of Clinical Nursing,* 15, 710-717.

Yiu, M. C. J., and Twinn, S. (2001). Determining the needs of Chinese parents during the hospitalization of their child diagnosed with cancer: An exploratory study. *Cancer Nursing,* 24(6), 483-489.

Zeltzer, L. K., Recklitis, C., Buchbinder, D., Zebrack, B., Casillas, J., Tsao, J. C. I., Lu, Q., and Krull, K. (2009). Psychological status in childhood cancer survivors: A report from the childhood cancer survivor study. *Journal of Clinical Oncology, 27*(14), 2396-2404.

In: Pediatric Cancer
Editor: William Li
ISBN: 978-1-61942-112-7

Chapter 6

DEVELOPING AND EVALUATING AN EMPOWERMENT PROGRAMME IN PROMOTING THE PSYCHOSOCIAL WELL-BEING AND QUALITY OF LIFE OF CHILDHOOD CANCER SURVIVORS: A PILOT STUDY

William H. C. Li
School of Nursing Studies, Li Ka Shing Faculty of Medicine
The University of Hong Kong, Hong Kong S.A.R., China

ABSTRACT

With advances in cancer screening and treatment, the survival rates for childhood cancer are higher than ever before. Yet, the course of treatment for cancer may lead to long term physical, emotional and psychosocial damage for children. Whilst much of the attention has focused on the physiological outcomes of cancer treatments in Hong Kong, the psychosocial well-being and quality of life of childhood cancer survivors have been disregarded or underestimated. Although various psychosocial interventions conducted in Western countries have shown beneficial effects on the psychosocial well-being of childhood cancer survivors, no similar intervention has been conducted in Hong Kong. Given to the different cultural background, it is uncertain whether the psychosocial interventions recommended by the Western literature can be appropriate for use in Hong Kong Chinese context. The aim of this chapter is to report a pilot study on developing and evaluating an empowerment programme for Hong Kong primary school students.

A pilot study of a randomized controlled trial, two-group pre-test and repeated post-test, between-subjects design was employed in two primary schools. A convenience sampling of 120 primary school students was recruited of whom 56 were randomly assigned to the experimental group participating in the empowerment programme and 64 to the control group receiving continuous assessment of their psychosocial well-being and quality of life. All the participants were asked to response to the Center for Epidemiologic Studies Depression Scale for Children, Rosenberg's Self-Esteem Scale and Pediatric Quality of Life Inventory across the three time periods: at the time of recruitment (T1: pre-intervention), and at six months (T2) and 12 months (T3) after starting the intervention.

The results of mixed between-within subjects ANOVA indicated that children in the experimental group reported statistically significant fewer depressive symptoms and higher self-esteem than children in the control group. The findings added further evidence that children who engaged in a healthy lifestyle, eating healthily and exercising regularly, reported fewer depressive symptoms and higher levels of self-esteem than those who did not engage in such a lifestyle. Furthermore, teaching children problem-solving and interpersonal skills, as well as how to cope with stress and adversity, it can enhance their psychosocial well-being and strengthen their resilience to psychological distress. Most importantly, this study has demonstrated the feasibility of implementing the empowerment programme in the Hong Kong Chinese context. The content, nature and duration of the empowerment programme were found to be acceptable by Hong Kong Chinese children and their parents. Therefore, it is anticipated that with some minor modifications, the empowerment programme can be used as an appropriate psychosocial interventions to promote psychosocial well-being and quality of life of Hong Kong Chinese childhood cancer survivors. In addition, health care professionals should set up a community supporting network for children with cancer and their family so that children can better combat with adverse psychosocial effects of cancer and its subsequent adverse treatment effects at every step of their long and difficult journey.

INTRODUCTION

As more children are surviving cancer than ever before, there is a growing awareness of the important of their emotional and psychosocial well-being. Previous cancer survivor studies revealed that quite a number of childhood cancer survivors developed chronic health problems in early adulthood, such as second malignancies, growth and endocrine dysfunction, and serious organ toxicities (Hudon, et al., 2003, Sharp, kinahan, Didwania, and Stolley, 2007). Most of these chronic health problems are considered late effects of the cancer treatments resulting from chemotherapy and radiation. However, childhood cancer survivors may not only at risk for medical adverse effects, their psychosocial well-being, self-esteem and quality of life may also severely affect as a result of their cancer and its therapy (Langeveld, et al., 2004). Previous study indicated that irradiation, chemotherapy, and surgical intervention may exert long-term effects on childhood cancer survivors' psychological outcomes, including anxiety and depression (Zeltzer, et al., 2009). Nevertheless, in Hong Kong, most attention has been drawn to the physiological care of childhood cancer survivors and has disregarded the importance of the late medical adverse effects on their psychosocial well-being.

Like most healthy children, childhood cancer survivors just want to grow up healthy and happy. Therefore, ensuring healthy psychosocial well-being in childhood cancer survivors, in particular enhancing their quality of life should be a prime concern of healthcare professionals (Chien, et al., 2003). Over the past decade, numerous Western studies have focused on developing and evaluating different psychosocial interventions for childhood cancer survivors (Andersen, Golden-Kreutz, Emery, and Debora, 2009; Hudson et al., 1998; Hudson, Tyc, Srivastava, Gattuso, Quargnenti, and Crom, 2002; Kazak, 2005). Interventions include psycho-educational, cognitive, behavioural and biological components have shown beneficial effects on psycho-social well-being of childhood cancer survivors. Yet, a review of the literature reveals that, so far, no similar study has been conducted in the Hong Kong. Because the cultural context in which Hong Kong Chinese children live is drastically different from that of Western children, the way that they view the nature and meaning of their illness will also differ considerably from those of Western children. Additionally, the ways which children use to cope with and respond to the illness may differ, which is susceptible to cultural differences (Li, 2009). Lazarus and Folkman (1984) point out that difference in the ways in which individuals cope may be expected to affect each person's response to a psychological intervention. Consequently, it is uncertain whether the psychosocial interventions proposed by Western studies are also effective for Hong Kong Chinese childhood cancer survivors. Given these issues, it is crucial to develop and evaluate appropriate psychosocial interventions for Hong Kong Chinese childhood survivors. First, however, understanding the cultural background, in particular the mental well-being of Hong Kong Chinese children is an essential prerequisite for the design of an appropriate psychosocial intervention to promote their psychosocial well-being and enhance their quality of life.

The Mental Well-Being of Hong Kong Chinese Children

Over the past two decades, Hong Kong has been undergoing a rapid socio-political transition with major changes in social and economic structure, traditional values, family structure and education curriculum. A comprehensive review of mental health of children revealed that there are some differences in the cognitive behaviour of Hong Kong Chinese children when compared with the Western counterparts (Wong and Tsoi, 1999). Hong Kong Chinese children generally lack creativity, and creative thinking when compared with Western children. This may have been influenced by Hong Kong's socio-cultural emphasis on obedience and social conformity, academic performance, inhibition of self-expression, and avoidance of being deviant or making mistakes (Tsoi and Pryde, 1999). A recent longitudinal study to examine the relationships between perceived parental psychological control and psychological well-being in Hong Kong Chinese children revealed that parental psychological control may inhibit the development of positive mental well-being and affect emotional life in children (Shek, 2007).

On the other hand, the family structure in Hong Kong has undergone significant changes, with traditional extended families have gradually been replaced by small nuclear families (Census and Statistics Department, 2007). Lam et al. (2004) claimed that the change from an extended to a nuclear family structure has had an impact on children's mental health. Because there are fewer siblings in a nuclear family, children are afforded more attention and tend to be over-protected by parents. In a study examining family functioning and psychological well being, school adjustment, and problem behaviour in Chinese children, Shek (2002) found that today's Hong Kong Chinese children are more vulnerable and less resilient to psychological distress compared to those of the previous generation.

Given to the specific cultural context in Hong Kong, it is uncertain whether the impact of cancer and its treatment on Chinese children is similar to that experienced by children in the West. Furthermore, the psychosocial interventions recommended by Western literature may not be appropriate for Hong Kong Chinese childhood cancer survivors. With these issues in mind, this chapter is a report of development and pilot testing the effectiveness of an empowerment programme in promoting the psychosocial well-being of Hong Kong Chinese children. The objectives of this chapter were:

1. To develop an empowerment programme for Hong Kong Chinese Children
2. To pilot test the effectiveness of the empowerment programme in minimizing depressive symptoms and enhancing the self-esteem and quality of life for Hong Kong Chinese children.
3. To identify implications for practice with the aims to promote psychosocial well-being and enhance the quality of life for Hong Kong Chinese childhood cancer survivors

Development of an Empowerment Programme for Hong Kong Chinese Children

To develop the programme, an advisory committee was set up which included the researcher, an assistant professor at a local university with considerable experience of conducting psychosocial interventions among children, two social workers from a Youth and Children Integrated Community Centre and two teachers with more than ten years' experience of teaching primary school children.

The Content and Rationales of Empowerment Programme

The programme content is based on evidence from previous literatures and expert opinion from the members of advisory committee. The major objectives of the empowerment programme were:

1. To promote awareness of the importance of positive mental health to primary school children
2. To equip primary school children with the knowledge and skills to cope with stress and adversity
3. To advocate a healthy lifestyle and empower primary school children to adopt it, in particular healthy eating and regular exercise, so as to promote their psychosocial well-being and strengthen their resilience to psychological distress

The content included teaching children how to face adversity, understand their emotions, develop positive thinking, develop positive values and attitudes toward life and lead a healthy lifestyle through eating healthy and exercising regularly. In addition, the empowerment programme contains workshops for teaching students problem solving and coping skills, interpersonal communication skills and relaxation exercises. The content of the empowerment programme is shown in Table 1.

Table 1. Content of the Empowerment Programme for Primary School Students

Date and time	Health Talks and Workshops
October 30 minutes 45 minutes	Health Education Talk (1) What is positive psycho-social well-being? Workshop (1) • Activities on knowing each others • Emotional expression
November 30 minutes 45 minutes	Health Talk (2) Importance of having regular physical activities and healthy eating Workshop (2) • Problem-solving skills and relaxation exercises
February 30 minutes 45 minutes	Health Education Talk (3) Understand what stress is and how it affects your health Workshop (3) Stress management skills and coping strategies
April 30 minutes 45 minutes	Health Education Talk (4) Develop positive thinking and attitude Workshop (4) Facing adversity
May 30 minutes 45 minutes	Health Education Talk (5) Communication skills Workshop (5) Social and interpersonal skills
July 09:00 to 16:00	Adventure-based Day Camp Objectives: enhancing children's social and interpersonal skills, problem-solving skills and self-esteem. Activities: games, play and adventure activities, group games and debriefing

* Remarks: Apart from attending education talks and workshops, participants in the experimental group were encouraged to join at least a one-hour's session of age appropriated physical leisure activities weekly, organized by and held in a nearby community centre every Saturday and Sunday.

It has been well documented that physical activity has beneficial effects on our physical well-being, particularly in relation to coronary heart diseases (WHO, 1995). There is also evidence to demonstrate that physical activity can also be effective in improving our mental well-being, for instance reduced state anxiety, resilience to stress, improved mood states and enhanced self-esteem (Fox, 1999). In addition, previous study showed that children who engaged in a healthy lifestyle, such as eating healthy and exercising regularly have less depressive symptoms and better emotional and physical health than those who do not engage in a healthy lifestyle (Lee, 2004). Yet, a large-scale surveillance conducted in 2003 to examine eating habits, exercise pattern, risk behaviours, violence behaviours and psychological well-being of school students revealed that majority of primary and secondary school students did not have the required healthy eating standard and less than 50% of the students performed regular exercises (CUHK's School of Public Health, 2003). The findings also revealed that those students who engaged in a healthy lifestyle, such as having healthy eating and regular exercises, had less depressive symptoms and better emotional than those who did not engage in a healthy lifestyle.

There are many reasons why a healthy lifestyle, in particular regular exercise, is vital to our psychosocial well-being. Physiological theories claim that the levels of neurotransmitters (endorphine, serotonin and norepinephrine) in the brain are elevated following acute exercise (Morgan, 1997). These chemical substances can help reduce anxiety, improve mood and ease depression. In addition, the changes of core body temperature during exercise may have a calming effect on the emotions. Behavioural theories also suggest that perception of mastery; self-worth and self-efficacy are associated with the completion of exercise (Landers and Arent, 2001).

Specially, social cognitive theory postulates that enhanced perceptions of capability, such as self-efficacy lead to improved psychological states (Bandura, 1986). In addition, psychoanalytic theories (Morgan, 1982) hold that regular physical activity is essential for children's growth and development, enhancing their ability to feel in control of their lives, and maintaining their mental ability to resist stress by altering the biochemical secretions in the brain. It is therefore believed that through helping children engage in healthy pursuits their mental well-being will be promoted.

Indeed, the content of the programme is quite comprehensive, and includes teaching schoolchildren how to cope with stress and strengthen their resilience to psychological distress. Such content has been frequently used in previous studies and was found to be most effective in promoting psychosocial well-being for young people than other treatment approaches (Hoagwood and Erwin, 1997).

Additionally, the content of the programme includes components of both problem- and emotion-focused interventions. Previous studies have found that patients receiving mixed-focused interventions have better psychological outcomes than those receiving either emotion- or problem- focused interventions alone (Li, Lopez and Lee, 2007; Martelli, Auerbach, Alexander and Mercuri,1987).

The proposed intervention protocol of the empowerment Programme was then sent for validation to a clinical psychologist at a community centre who had experience of working with children. The psychologist was asked to assess the dosage of the intervention in terms of the amount, frequency, duration and breadth. This measure ensured that the intervention delivered was adequate for quality assessment and the management of outcomes, such as depressive symptoms, self-esteem and quality of life.

TESTING THE EFFECTIVENESS OF AN EMPOWERMENT PROGRAMME FOR HONG KONG CHINESE CHILDREN

Method

Design

To test the effectiveness of the empowerment programme, a randomized controlled trial, two-group pre-test and repeated post-test, between-subjects design was employed in two primary schools. We targeted to recruit 60 children from each primary school in this pilot study.

The method of simple complete randomization was adopted and performed in each school. We put two sealed opaque envelopes in a box, with one labelled experimental and another labelled control. Each parent was asked to draw one envelop from the box for each child to determine group assignment.

Another sealed opaque envelop with the same group assignment being drawn was then put back in the box again before the next assignment.

Sample

Primary school students from two schools in one of the largest public housing estates in Hong Kong who met the study's inclusion criteria were invited to participate in the study. The inclusion criteria were the following: (1) Hong Kong Chinese primary 5 and 6 students (5th and 6th grade); and (2) able to speak Cantonese and read Chinese. Children with identified cognitive and learning problems were excluded. A convenience sampling of 120 children was recruited (60 from each school), of whom 56 were randomly assigned to the experimental group and 64 to the control group.

There are reasons for selecting primary 5 and 6 students as the target population. Such children are at the stage of a complex transitional period - with reference to the theory of social development (Erikson, 1963), they have entered the stage of 'Fidelity', which is dominated by role confusion, searching for a personality identity and being influenced by peers. Additionally, primary 5 and 6 students will experience the contextual shift from primary school to secondary school, with different academic and social expectations. Within these contexts, they are psychologically vulnerable and health promotion is crucial in empowering them to maintain mental well-being.

Intervention

Using the method of simple randomization, 60 students from each school were randomly assigned into the experimental and control groups, after the pre-test baseline measurements were taken. In the control group, students underwent continuous assessment of their psychosocial well-being and quality of life throughout an academic year.

In the experimental group, children were invited to participate in the empowerment programme, which was implemented in their schools's assembly hall on Saturday morning, two identical programmes being implemented in the two schools. The empowerment programme consisted of five half-day sessions (around 75 minutes per session) and a day camp at the end of the academic year. Each session comprised health education talks and a workshop. The talks were addressed to both children and parents, while the workshops were limited to children only (see Table 1). The empowerment programme was implemented by health care professionals and social workers throughout a school academic year. The advantage of using a multidisciplinary approach is that each discipline can be strengthened and complemented each other. Furthermore, a multidisciplinary approach encourages knowledge transfer and enhances problem-solving abilities between disciplines.

Additionally, it facilitates the development of infrastructure, to ensure a network can deliver and sustain a programme. All education talks and workshops were held at the assembly hall of schools on Saturday morning. The teaching mole in the workshops was interactive, and incorporated role-play, games and a variety of play activities. Apart from attending talks and workshops, participants in the experimental group were encouraged to join at least one-hour's session of age-appropriate physical leisure activities weekly, organised by and held in a nearby community centre every Saturday and Sunday. Examples of such activities were table tennis, badminton, basketball, volleyball, football, a variety of chess games and Chinese billiards.

Measurements

Demographic Data Sheet

A demographic data sheet was used to document children's demographic characteristics. In addition, parents' education attainment was also documented, which can provide indirect information that reflects the socio-economic status of a family.

The Center for Epidemiologic Studies Depression Scale for Children (CES-DC)

The CES-DC comprises 20 fully standardized items to evaluate depressive symptoms. The items consist of short and simple statements in the first person about the emotional, cognitive and behaviour related components of depressiveness. All items are evaluated on a four-point Likert scale in relation to their incidence during the last week, which were scored from 0 to 3 (0 = "not at all," 1 = "a little," 2 = "sometimes," 3 = "a lot"), with total possible scores ranging from 0 to 60, with higher scores indicating greater symptomatology. The cut-off point is fixed at 16. A score of 16 or greater indicates an individual demonstrating some depressive symptoms. The psychometric properties of the CES-DC have been empirically tested (Barkmann, Erhart, and Schulte-Markwort, 2008), showing adequate internal consistency reliability, good concurrent validity, and excellent construct validity. The results of confirmatory factor analysis showed that there are four factors underlying the CES-DC, which is congruent with hypothesized configuration of the factor structure of the CES-D proposed by Radloff (1977). The four-factor version of the CES-DC is considered to have good factorial validity and stability across age (Barkmann et al., 2008).

The psychometric properties of the Chinese version of the CES-DC have been empirically tested (Li, Chung, and Ho, 2010), showing adequate internal consistency reliability good content validity and appropriate convergent and discriminant validity. Confirmatory factor analysis added further evidence of the construct validity of the scale.

Rosenberg's Self-Esteem Scale (RSES)

The RSES was designed to measure self-esteem as a global disposition (Rosenberg 1965) and has been widely used with adolescents (Byrne, 2000; Kim, 2003) and children (Phillips, Bodfield, Woodthorpe, and Gimsley, 2008). The RSES consists of 10 items, an example being 'I am able to do things as well as most other people'. Responses are rated using a 4-point Likert scale ranging from 1 (strongly disagree) to 4 (strongly agree), with total possible scores ranging from 10 to 40. Higher scores indicate higher levels of self-esteem.

The Chinese version of the RSES has been used with children (Society for Community Organization, 2004). The results suggest that the Chinese version of the RSES can be used as a self-report assessment tool in measuring self-esteem of Chinese children.

Pediatric Quality of Life Inventory (PedsQL)

The PedsQL is a widely used scale to assess the health-related quality of life among children and adolescents between the age of 2 and 18 years (Varni, Burwinkle, Katz, Meeske, and Dickinson, 2002). It can be applied to both healthy children and paediatric patient population. The instrument consists of 23 items grouped into 4 subscales: physical functioning (8 items), emotional functioning (5 items), social functioning (5 items) and school functioning (5 items). Participants were asked how much of a problem has been experienced over the last month, which were scored from 0 to 4 (0 = never a problem, 1 = almost never a problem; 2= sometimes a problem, 3= often a problem, 4 = almost always a problem). The items are then reverse-scored and linearly transformed to a 0-100 scale (0 = 100, 1 = 75, 2 = 50, 3 = 25, 4 = 0). The scale scores were obtained by summing the items and dividing by the number of items of the scale. After transformation, scores range from 0 to 100, with higher scores indicating better health-related qualify of life. The psychometric properties of the Chinese version of the PedsQL have been empirically tested (Chan, Chow, and Lo, 2005). Results suggest that the Chinese version of the PedsQL can be used as a reliable and valid measure of health-related quality of life in Chinese paediatric research and clinical application.

Study Procedure

Study approval was obtained by the ethics committee of a local university. The principal of each school was fully informed about the study's purpose, nature, design, and duration. Written consent was obtained from the parents after they were told the purpose of the study. They were given the option to participate or refuse their child's involvement in the study. The children were also invited to put their names on a special children's assent form and told that their participation was voluntary and were assured of the confidentiality of the study. Data collection was divided into three phases: at the time of recruitment (T1: pre-intervention), and at six months (T2) and 12 months (T3) after starting the intervention. All participants were asked to respond to the Chinese version of the CES-DC, the RSES, and the PedsQL.

Data Analysis

The Statistical Package for Social Sciences (SPSS: Version 18.0; SPSS Inc., Chicago, IL, USA) for Windows was used for data analysis. The homogeneity of the experimental and control groups were assessed by using inferential statistics (independent *t*-test and χ^2). Descriptive statistics were used to calculate the mean scores and standard deviation of different scales. Mixed between-within subjects ANOVA (split-plot ANOVA) was used to determine whether the empowerment programme was effective in minimizing depressive symptoms and enhancing self-esteem and quality of life of school children.

Results

Information on the demographic and baseline characteristics of the experimental and control groups is presented in Table 2.

The results revealed that the experimental and control groups were similar with respect to the age and gender of children, education attainment of parents, and baseline depressive symptoms, self-esteem and quality of life of children, suggesting a high level of homogeneity of variance between these two groups in this study. The mean scores and standard deviation of the depressive symptoms, self-esteem and quality of life across the three time periods are presented in Table 3.

Table 2. Comparison of experimental and control groups on demographic and baseline characteristics (n = 120)

	n (%)		p[a]
	Experimental (*n* = 56)	Control (*n* = 64)	
Gender of Children			
Male	29 (51.8)	34 (53.1)	0.96 ns
Female	27 (48.2)	30 (46.9)	
Education attainment (parents)			
Primary	7 (12.5)	6 (9.4)	0.92 ns
Lower secondary	19 (33.9)	21 (32.8)	
Upper secondary	24 (42.9)	29 (45.3)	
Tertiary	6 (10.7)	8 (12.5)	
	M (S.D.)		p[a]
	Experimental (*n* = 56)	Control (*n* = 64)	
Age of children	11.4(2.3)	11.8 (2.4)	0.88 ns
Depressive symptoms	13.66 (6.8)	12.98 (6.3)	0.70 ns
Self-esteem	28.36 (6.9)	27.95 (6.5)	0.74 ns
Quality of life	70.4 (14.4)	71.0 (14.4)	0.78 ns

ns: not significant at $p > 0.05$.
[a] Group comparisons t-test for continuous and $\chi 2$ for nominal and categorical variables.

The results of mixed between-within subjects ANOVA on the scores of the depressive symptoms scores, self-esteem and quality of life across the three time periods are shown in Table 4. The results indicated that children in the experimental group reported statistically significant fewer depressive symptoms and higher self-esteem than children in the control group. Using the commonly used guidelines proposed by Cohen (1992), the eta squared of 0.01, 0.06, and 0.14 are typically interpreted as small, moderate, and large effect sizes respectively. The results suggest moderate intervention effect sizes. Post-hoc test, using Tukey procedure, confirmed that the differences in depressive symptoms scores between groups were statistically significant at both six months (T2) and twelve months (T3) after starting the intervention. Besides, there was a statistically significant different in self-esteem scores between groups at twelve months (T3) after starting the intervention. Nevertheless, the results of mixed between-within subjects ANOVA showed that there was no statistically significant difference in children's quality of life between the experimental and control groups at T2 and T3.

Table 3. The mean scores and standard deviations for depressive symptoms, self-esteem and quality of life in children between two groups across three time periods ($n = 120$)

	Mean (S.D.)		
	Experimental ($n = 56$)	Control ($n = 64$)	Total ($n = 120$)
Depressive symptoms:			
T1	13.66 (6.84)	12.98 (6.34)	13.30 (6.52)
T2	10.14 (6.49)	13.23 (6.56)	11.79 (5.97)
T3	9.77 (5.82)	12.92 (6.44)	11.45 (5.83)
Self-esteem:			
T1	28.36 (6.95)	27.95 (6.45)	28.14 (6.66)
T2	29.52 (6.94)	27.77 (6.19)	28.58 (6.58)
T3	30.59 (6.82)	28.08 (6.33)	29.25 (6.66)
Quality of life			
T1	70.38 (14.39)	70.95 (14.37)	70.68 (14.24)
T2	71.97 (14.55)	70.34 (14.27)	71.10 (14.07)
T3	73.96 (14.96)	71.15 (13.92)	72.46 (14.37)

Notes: T1 = Data collection at the time of recruitment (before intervention); T2 = Data collection at 6 months after starting the intervention, T3 = Data collection at 12 months after starting the intervention.

Table 4. The results of mixed between-within subjects ANOVA on depressive symptoms, self-esteem and quality of life scores in children across three time periods (n = 120)across the three time periods (n = 120)

	Depression symptoms			Self-esteem			Quality of life		
	F-value	p-value	Eta Squared	F-value	p-value	Eta Squared	F-value	p-value	Eta Squared
Time Effect	34.69	0.00*	0.23	22.51	0.00*	0.22	2.68	0.09	0.04
Interaction Effect	37.38	0.00*	0.24	20.31	0.00*	0.19	0.78	0.56	0.03
Intervention Effect	3.22	0.03*	0.06	3.01	0.04*	0.04	0.06	0.81	0.02

Notes: * Significant at p <0.05.

Discussion

Notwithstanding survival rates are higher than ever before as a result of new technology and breakthroughs in cancer treatment, childhood cancer survivors are at risk for medical and psychosocial late effects of the cancer treatment resulting from chemotherapy toxicities, radiation, or secondary cancers. The late effects may even last for many years after completion of therapy, severely affecting children's psychosocial well-being and quality of life. It is thus crucial to develop and evaluate interventions that can help ease the burden of sequelae of cancer and its treatment and provide psychosocial support for childhood cancer survivors at every step of their long and difficult journey. The aim of this study was to test the effectiveness of the empowerment programme in minimizing depressive symptoms and enhancing the self-esteem and quality of life for Hong Kong Chinese children. Once the effectiveness of the empowerment programme is confirmed, health care professionals may consider using this programme to promote psychosocial well-being and quality of life of Hong Kong Chinese childhood cancer survivors.

Effect of the Empowerment Programme on Children's Depressive Symptoms and Self-esteem

The results of mixed between-within subjects ANOVA on the depressive symptoms and self-esteem scores indicated that there were statistically significant main effects for time in the scores of depressive symptoms and self-esteem, suggesting a change in the depressive symptoms and self-esteem between two groups across the three time periods. Yet there were statistically significant interaction effects between the time and intervention, indicating that the changes in depressive symptoms and self-esteem of children over the different times were dissimilar between the experimental and control groups. The results showed that children in the experimental group reported statistically significant fewer depressive symptoms and higher level of self-esteem than children in the control group.

The findings are consistent with previous studies (CUHK's School of Public Health, 2003; Fox, 1999; Lee, 2004), showing that children who engaged in a healthy lifestyle, eating healthily and exercising regularly, reported fewer depressive symptoms and higher self-esteem than those children who did not engage in such a lifestyle. In addition, the findings added further evidence that teaching children problem-solving and interpersonal skills, as well as how to cope with stress and adversity, can enhance their psychosocial well-being and strengthen their resilience to psychological distress.

The results showed that there were statistically significant differences in depressive symptoms between the groups at T2 and T3. However, only a statistically significant difference in self-esteem scores between groups was found at T3. One possible reason is that, because of the transitory nature of depressive symptoms, they may vary in intensity, fluctuating from time to time as a result of exposure to different situations. However, unlike depressive symptom, self-esteem is moderately stable over time and change may therefore tale longer to appear within a person.

Effect of the Empowerment Programme on Children's Quality of Life

The mean scores for quality of life among children in the experimental group were higher than in the control group. Nevertheless, the results of mixed between-within subjects ANOVA indicated that there were no statistically significant main effect for time, and interaction effect. The findings suggest that the quality of life of children in both groups did not change across the three different time periods, regardless of the type of intervention. Additionally, there was no statistically significant difference between the experimental and control groups in quality of life. One possible explanation lies in the difficulty of determining whether the quality of life of healthy school children could be expected to respond to the empowerment programme. It had a more precise effect on minimizing depressive symptoms and enhancing self-esteem for children, while the outcome measures of quality of life might be less responsive to the intervention. Another possible reason is that the relationship between the programme and children's quality of life might have been affected by the limited size of the sample when using the PedsQL. It would therefore be interesting to see if further studies using larger samples could find a significant relationship between the empowerment programme and children's quality of life.

There was a considerable amount of positive feedback from children receiving the empowerment programme. One of their comments was as follows:

> 'Before joining this programme, I used to do things without confidence and had the feeling that I was not as good as my peers. After this programme, I have taken a positive attitude towards myself, realising that I am able to do things just as well as most other people. Additionally, I no longer get easily frustrated as I did before. Although some tasks are challenging for me, I can cooperate with others to handle them.'

Implications for Practice

It has been well documented that cancer and its treatments have a tremendous impact on the psychosocial well-being and quality of life of childhood cancer survivors. It is therefore essential for healthcare professionals to develop and evaluate appropriate interventions with the aim of promoting psychosocial well-being for these children. The most important implications for practice from this study relate to the determination of the effectiveness of the empowerment programme in promoting psychosocial well-being for Hong Kong Chinese children. Furthermore, this study has demonstrated the feasibility of implementing the empowerment programme in the Hong Kong Chinese context. The content, nature and duration of the empowerment programme were acceptable to Hong Kong Chinese children and their parents. Indeed, some evidence exists to support that advocate a healthy lifestyle for childhood cancer survivors can help modify the evolution of the late psychosocial adverse effects of cancer and its treatment (Clarke and Eiser, 2007; Nathan, et al., 2009). In addition, through teaching childhood cancer survivors problem-solving, and interpersonal skills, facing adversity, developing positive values and attitude and how to cope with stress, it will strengthen their resilience against the late-emerging adverse psychosocial effects of cancer and its treatment. Therefore, it is anticipated that with some minor modifications the empowerment programme can be used as an appropriate psychosocial interventions to promote psychosocial well-being and enhance quality of life of Hong Kong Chinese childhood cancer survivors. Most importantly, health care professionals should take one step forward to extend beyond their role in collaborating with education sectors and school social workers to provide psychosocial education and support to childhood cancer survivors in a multidisciplinary approach. Specifically, health care professionals should set up a community supporting network for childhood cancer survivors so that they can better combat with adverse psychosocial effects of cancer and its treatment and are able to go on their journey with renewed hope and faith.

Study Limitation

The use of convenience sampling limits the ability of this study to generalize the results. Another limitation is that this study did not include a process evaluation in assessing the effectiveness of the empowerment programme notwithstanding it is important to identify the strengths and limitations of the new model of care delivery from the participants' perspectives. Indeed a process evaluation can help understand the important ingredient of the intervention and improve the future presentations of the intervention. Most importantly, a process evaluation can help optimize the quality and effectiveness of a newly developed intervention, as well as to determine whether the intervention is feasible and acceptable to both health care professionals and participants. Therefore, it is recommended future study should include a process evaluation on the effectiveness, feasibility and appropriateness of the empowerment programme.

Conclusion

Despite its possible limitation, this study has addressed a gap in the literature by developing an appropriate and effectiveness empowerment programme to enhance mental well-being for Hong Kong Chinese children. The findings of this study have adduced further evidence of the importance of advocating a healthy lifestyle in promoting children's psychosocial well-being. It is anticipate that this empowerment programme can also be used to promote psychosocial well-being and quality of life of Hong Kong Chinese childhood cancer survivors.

REFERENCES

Andersen, B. L., Golden-Kreutz, D. M., Emery, C. F., and Debora, L. T. (2009). Biobehavioral Intervention for Cancer Stress: Conceptualization, Components, and Intervention Strategies. *Cognitive and Behavioral Practice,* 16(3), 253-265.

Bandura, A. (1986). *Social foundations of thought and action: a social cognitive theory*. New Jersey: Prentice-Hall.

Barkmann, C., Erhart, M., and Schulte-Markwort, M. (2008). The German version of the Centre for Epidemiological Studies Depression Scale for Children: psychometric evaluation in a population-based survey of 7 to 17 years old children and adolescents – results of the BELLA study. *European Child and Adolescent Psychiatry,* 17, 116-124.

Byrne, B. (2000). Relationship between anxiety, fear, self-esteem and coping strategies in adolescence. *Adolescence,* 35(137), 215-301.

Census and Statistics Department. (2007). *2006 Population By-census. Summary results*. Hong Kong Special Administrative Region, People's Republic of China.

Chan, L. F. P., Chow, S. M. K, and Lo, S. K. (2005). Preliminary validation of the Chinese version of the pediatric quality of life inventory. *International Journal of Rehabilitation Research*, 28(3), 219-227.

Chien, L. Y., Lo, L. H., Chen C. J., Chen, Y. C., Chiang, C. C, and Chao, Y. M. Y. (2003). Quality of life among primary caregivers of Taiwanese children with brain tumor. *Cancer Nursing, 26*, 305-311.

Clarke, S. A., and Eiser, C. (2007). Health behaviours in childhood cancer survivors: A systematic review. *European Journal of Cancer, 43*, 1373-1384.

Cohen, J. (1992). A power primer. *Psychological Bulletin, 112*, 155-159.

CUHK's School of Public Health *(2003).* Tsuen Wan students' health need improvement-Regular exercises and healthy eating lower emotional problem. Retrieved March 8, 2009, from Web site: http://www.cuhk.edu.hk/med/hep/chi/research/reports/c_tsuenwan.htm.

Erikson, E. (1963). *Childhood and society*. (2nd Ed.). New York: W.W. Norton and Company.

Fox, K. R. (1999). The influence of physical activity on mental well-being. *Public Health Nutrition,* 2(3a), 411-418.

Hoagwood, K., and Erwin, H. D. (1997). Effectiveness of school-based mental health services for children: A 10-year research review. *Journal of Child and Family Studies, 33*(6), 435-51.

Hudson, M. M., Hinds, P. S., Tyc, V., Gattuso, J., Quargnenti, A., Srivastava, D. K., Crom, D. B. and Mason, C. (1998). An educational intervention to improve health knowledge and behavior in childhood cancer survivors. *Journal of Pediatric Oncology Nursing,* 15(2), 112-113.

Hudson, M. M., Mertens, A. C., Yasui, Y., Hobbie, W., Chen, H., Gurney, J. G., Yeazel, M., Reckitis, C. J., Marina, N., Robison, L. R., and Oeffinger K.C. (2003). Health status of adult long-term survivors of childhood cancer: A report from the Childhood Cancer Survivor Study. *Journal of the American Medical Association,* 290, 1583-339.

Hudson, M. M., Tyc, V. L., Srivastava, D. K., Gattuso, J., Quargnenti, A. and Crom, D. B. (2002). Multi-component behavioral intervention to promote health protective behaviors in childhood cancer survivors: the protect study. *Medical and Pediatric Oncology,* 39, 2-11.

Kazak, A. E. (2005). Evidence-based interventions for survivors of childhood cancer and their families. *Journal of Pediatric Psychology,* 30(1), 29-39.

Kim, Y. H. (2003). Correlation of mental health problems with psychological constructs in adolescence: final results from a 2-year study. *International Journal of Nursing Studies,* 40, 115-124.

Lam, T. H., Stewart, S. M., Yip, P. S. F., Leung, G. M., Ho, L. M., Ho, D. S.Y., et al. (2004). Suicidality and cultural values among Hong Kong adolescents. *Social Science and Medicine, 58,* 487-498.

Landers, D. M., and Arent, S. M. (2001). Physical activity and mental health. In R. N. Singer, H. A. Hausenblas, and C. M. Janelle (EDS.), *Handbook of sport psychology (pp747-765).* (2nd ed.) New York: Wiley.

Langeveld, N. E., Grootenhuis, M. A., Voute, P. A., Haan, R. J., and Bos, C. V. D. (2004). Quality of life, self-esteem and worries in young adult survivors of childhood cancer. *Psycho-Oncology, 13,* 867-881.

Lazarus, R. S., and Folkman, S. (1984). Stress, appraisal, and coping. New York: Springer.

Lee, A. (2004). Helping students to adopt healthy lifestyle and positive youth development through school setting: Hong Kong experience of health promoting school. *Hong Kong Journal of Paediatric, 9,* 325-28.

Li, H. C. W., Chung, O. K. J. and Ho, K. Y. E. (2010) Psychometric Testing of the Chinese version of the Center for Epidemiologic Studies Depression Scale for Children. *Journal of Advanced Nursing, 66(11), 2582-2591.*

Li, H. C. W., Lopez, V. and Lee, T. L. I. (2007). Effects of Preoperative Therapeutic Play on Outcomes of School-age Children Undergoing Day Surgery. *Research in Nursing and Health, 30,* 320-332.

Li, W. H. C. (2009). The Importance of Incorporating Cultural Issues into Nursing Interventions for Chinese Populations. In W.T. Chien (Eds). *Strategies in evaluation of complex health care interventions for people with physical or mental health issues*, New York: Nova Biomedical Book.

Martelli, M. F., Auerbach, S. M., Alexander, J., and Mercuri, L. G. (1987). Stress Management in the health care setting: Matching interventions with patient coping styles. *Journal of Consulting and Clinical Psychology, 55*, 201-207.

Morgan, W. P. (1982). Psychological effects of exercise. *Behavioral Medicine Update*, *4*, 25-30.

Morgan, W. P. (1997). Physical activity and mental health. Washington, DC: Talyer and Francis.

Nathan, P. C., Ford, J. S., Henderson, T. O., Hudson, M. M., Emmons, J. N., Casillas, J. N., et al. (2009). Health behaviours, medical care, and interventions to promote healthy living in childhood cancer survivor study cohort. *Journal of Clinical Oncology,* 27(14), 2363-2373.

Phillips, D., Bodfield, E., Woodthorpe, K., and Gimsley, M. (2008). Exploring the impact of group work and mentoring for multiple heritage children's self-esteem, well-being and behaviour. *Health and Social Care in the Community,* 16(3), 310-321.

Radloff, L. S. (1977). A CES-D scale: A self-report depression scale for research in the general population. *Applied Psychological Measurement,* 1, 385-401.

Rosenberg, M. (1965). *Society and Adolescent Self-image.* Princeton University Press, Princeton.

Sharp, L. K., Kinahan, K. E., Didwania, A., and Stolley, M. (2007). Quality of life in adult survivors of childhood cancer. *Journal of Pediatric Oncology Nursing,* 24(4), 220-226.

Shek, D. T. L. (2002). Family functioning and psychological well being, school adjustment, and problem behavior in Chinese adolescents with and without economic disadvantage. *Journal of Genetic Psychology, 163*, 497-502.

Shek, D. T. L. (2007). A longitudinal study of perceived parental psychological control and psychological well-being in Chinese adolescents in Hong Kong. *Journal of Clinical Psychology, 63*(1), 1-22.

Society for Community Organization. (2004). Today's Children. Future of Hong Kong: A survey report. Society for Community Organization.

Tsoi, M. M., and Pryde, N. A. (1999). Hong Kong's children: overview and conclusion. In N. A. Pryde and M. M Tsoi (EDS.), *Hong Kong's Children: our past, their future* (pp. 573-647). Hong Kong: Centre of Asian Studies, the University of Hong Kong.

Varni, J. W., Burwinkle, T. M., Katz, E. R., Meeske, K., and Dickinson, P. (2002). The PedsQL™ in pediatric cancer: Reliability and validity of the pediatric quality of life inventory™ generic core scale, multidimensional fatigue scale and cancer module. *Cancer, 94*(7), 2090-2106.

Wong, C. K., and Tsoi, M. M. (1999). Mental health of Hong Kong Children. In N.A. Pryde and M.M. Tsoi (EDS.), *Hong Kong's Children: our past, their future* (pp. 153-220). Hong Kong: Centre of Asian Studies, the University of Hong Kong.

World Health Organization (1995). Exercise for health. WHO/FIMS Committee on physical activity for health. *Bulletin of the World Health Organization,* 73(2), 135-6.

Zeltzer, L. K., Recklitis, C., Buchbinder, D., Zebrack, B., Casillas, J., Tsao, J. C. I., Lu, Q., and Krull, K. (2009). Psychological status in childhood cancer survivors: A report from the childhood cancer survivor study. *Journal of Clinical Oncology, 27*(14), 2396-2404.

In: Pediatric Cancer
Editor: William Li
ISBN: 978-1-61942-112-7

Chapter 7

PSYCHOSOCIAL SUPPORT FOR PARENTS OF CHILDREN WITH CANCER

Sau-ying Chiu[1] and Eva K. Y. Ho[2]
[1]Department of Paediatrics and Aldolescent Medicine
Queen Mary Hospital, Hong Kong S.A.R., China
[2]School of Nursing, Li Ka Shing Faculty of Medicine
The University of Hong Kong, Hong Kong S.A.R., China

ABSTRACT

Cancer is a life-threatening disease. The physical and psychological well-being of children with cancer is detrimentally influenced by the disease. It is not only the children who suffer from the disease as cancer also exerts negative influences on the patients' families. A review of the literature reveals that the parents who have children with cancer carry heavy burdens of care and responsibility. However, there are only few studies that discuss the life experience of the parents who have children with cancer. In this chapter, we will explore different coping mechanisms, hospital and community resources that are being utilized by parents who have children with cancer in eastern countries, in particular, Hong Kong.

Study: The objective of the study was to explore the life experience of parents who have chidren with cancer. For the purpose of this study, six mothers who are the primary caregivers were specifically selected from a paediatric oncology ward of a hospital. A semi-structured interview was conducted with each participant by a research nurse in the clinical area.

The results of the study showed that parents adopted emotion focused coping strategies in dealing with challenges. They were influenced by the fatalism and concept of a sense of personal honour. In addition, they also adopted problem focused coping strategies in order to control the situation. Different interventions which include counseling services, patient education, parent support group, assisting them to mobilize social support and providing spiritual support should be implemented in the clinical setting. It is essential for nurses to understand the coping strategies being utilized by parents, so as to design and evaluate appropriate nursing interventions that can enhance parents' abilities to cope with the challenges.

INTRODUCTION

Cancer is a life-threatening disease. Children who have cancer are overwhelmed by the invasive medical treatments, lengthy hospitalizations and frequent out-patient follow-ups. The physical and psychological well-being of children with cancer is detrimentally influenced by the disease. It is not only the children who suffer from the disease as cancer also exerts negative influences on the patients' families (Karak and Nachman, 1991). A review of the literature reveals that the parents who have children with cancer carry heavy burdens of care and responsibility. Indeed, parents are usually shocked when their children are newly diagnosed with cancer. The parents may feel helpless in managing the situation since some of them are lacking in medical knowledge related to the care of their children, while some parents find it difficult to strike a balance between the roles of being a caregiver and being a breadwinner. Because of the stress resulting from the child's illness, families may develop other problems such as financial difficulties and marital conflicts. On the other hand, parents are given hope that the childhood cancer can be treated and have some possibility of being cured; at the same time they also understand the fact that their children may be killed by the disease. The uncertainty of the prognosis causes parents to face a considerable level of anxiety and frustration during the years of treatment and perhaps the years beyond the last check-up. Therefore, families which have children with cancer must rearrange their routines, so as to cope with the new challenges. In this chapter, we will explore different coping mechanisms and hospital and community resources that are being utilized by parents who have children with cancer in eastern countries, in particular, Hong Kong.

LAZARUS STRESS-COPING MODEL

The Lazarus Stress-Coping Model serves as a guide for this study. Coping can be viewed as a process in the transaction of the individual and a stressor. It includes the cognitive and behavioral effort to manage the demands that are appraised as taxing or exceeding the resources of the individual (Folkmann and Lazarus, 1984). There are eight coping strategies, which are *confrontation, distancing, self-controlling, seeking social support, accepting responsibility, escape-avoidance, planful problem solving* and *positive appraisal* (personal growth, spirituality) (Taylor, 1995).

Coping is also classified as either problem focused or emotion focused (Lazarus and Folkman, 1984). Problem focused coping is directed at controlling the stressor to reduce or eliminate its stressfulness. It uses a problem solving process by defining the problem, generating alternative solutions, weighting the alternatives in terms of costs and benefits, choosing among them and implementing the selected solution. There are two coping strategies in the category of problem focused coping: seeking social support, and planful problem solving. Seeking social support is a coping strategy that describes a person defining himself or herself as an individual who needs to seek help from formal or informal sources (Barker, 2007). Planful problem solving is a coping strategy that involves effort and analytic skill to manage the stressful event in order to minimize its negative impact on their daily lives (Lambert and Lambert, 2008).

Unlike the problem focused coping, emotion focused coping is directed at controlling the emotional responses associated with the stressor. It aims to prevent people from becoming overwhelmed by negative emotions and engaging in actions to solve the problem. There are six different coping strategies within the category of emotion focused coping: confrontation; self control; distancing; escape and avoidance; positive appraisal; and accepting responsibility. Each of these six coping strategies are described as follows: (1) *confrontation*, which describes a person using hostility or aggressiveness to manage the stressful event; (2) *distancing*, which focuses on a person detaching himself or herself from a stressful environment thus minimizing the importance of the stressful event; (3) *self control*, which focuses on regulating personal emotions and actions; (4) *accepting responsibility*, which describes a person recognizing his or her role in controlling the stressful event; (5) *positive appraisal*, which describes a person giving a positive meaning to a stressful event; and (6) *escape and avoidance*, by which means a person is able to avoid the problem by using the method of denial and withdrawal.

Problem-focused coping and emotion-focused coping are often employed concurrently. However, we are more likely to choose problem-focused coping if we consider the stressor can be managed. Conversely, we tend to rely on emotion focused coping if we find it difficult to manage the stressful events (Sheridan and Radmacher, 1992).

COPING MECHANISM UTILIZED BY PARENTS

The purpose of this study was to explore the coping strategies utilized by parents in caring the children with cancer. Careful assessment of coping processes is necessary for the nurses to design appropriate interventions that can reduce primary caregivers' stress, bolster their coping mechanisms, and help them to regain self-confidence in caring their children.

Six mothers who have children newly diagnosed with cancer were interviewed to explore their life experiences. Approval for the study was obtained from the hospital ethical committee. Written consent was obtained from mothers after they were told the purpose of the study. The mothers were informed that they had right to withdraw from the study at any time and were assured of the confidentiality of the study.

In the study, we found that those mothers adopted a range of coping strategies which contain a lot of similarities. Both emotion focused and problem focused coping strategies were employed by them to cope with the challenges.

1. Emotion Focused Coping

1.1. Escape-Avoidance

The mothers reported that they could not accept the bad news in the initial phase. Therefore, escape-avoidanc was found to be an effective way for them to cope with the intense uncomfortable feelings, such as fear, grief or guit, during this brief period.

Here is a quote of an interviewed parent:

> 'When doctor told me the diagnosis (of my daughter), I didn't believe it. I was sure the result was wrong. ...Impossible ... I didn't know how to say it.' [Mother A.]

Although escape-avoidance is considered as a primitive or immature coping strategy, it serves an important protective function in the initial phase of adaptation to life-threatening illness. It allows time for an individual to 'regroup' and face the challenges (Hamburg, and Adam, 1967; Hackett and Weisman, 1967; cited in Rowland, 1990). However, it is essential for the health care professionals to differentiate a normal period of escape-avoidance coping from an abnormal period of escape-avoidance coping.

In addition, sharing feeling among the mothers was not explicit. They avoided sharing their feeling to others. Some mothers would hide their feeling, and resolve it by themselves. Besides, they disliked sympathy from others. They were afraid that other people may attribute the disease to be infections or sin. The stigmatization of cancer hinders those mothers from sharing their feeling to others. Accepting help from others may be viewed as admitting the failure in their commitment (Hull 1992).

Here is a quote of an interviewed parent:

> 'I don't want to let other know.... Tell other that my daughter has such a disease. ... They will think that I have done something wrong,... not good... maybe your daughter is infectious ... So I don't contact them by myself.' [Mother D]

Those mothers stated they were more willing to tell the others about the cancer diagnosis of their children after the brief period. However, the mothers still seldom involved their friends and relatives, since they might lack of time and the empathetic feeling.

Here are the quotes from interviewed mothers:

> 'I feel they don't understand me. Our mood is different.... They can't empathize with you. ... They don't know what you are thinking.' [Mother D]

> 'My son gets sick, just like I get sick. My friends want to visit me, but they can't come (because of the hospital regulation). I completely loss the contact (with my friend), even (can't) chat on the phone, because I am very busy to care my son.' [Mother C]

Some mothers wanted to share their feeling with their spouse and the health care professionals.

Here are the quotes from interviewed mothers:

> 'When my daughter's condition is critical, we cries but we (wife and husband) are hand in hand to face all the difficulties.' [Mother D]

> 'I am willing to talk about the whole process (my son critical condition in ICU). After talking, I feel better. [Mother C]

> 'The doctor and nurse here, (they) know us, I could express my grievance.' [Mother F]

Therefore, health care professionals should address the parents' intense emotional responses by active listening and counseling. Building mutual trust between the parents and health care professional are essential. Nurses should allay the patient's anxiety, fear before delivering any patient education.

Parents are also given relevant booklets and pamphlets which can assist them to understand some background information of the illness. At the same time, parents are visited by other parents whose children have recovered from cancer. The visits may instill sense of hope for the parents, and boost up their confidence to get through the cancer journey.

2. Problem Focused Coping

2.1. Information Seeking

Parents who have children with cancer would also employ problem focused coping strategies, which are planful problem solving and seeking social support.

Indeed, Felton and Revenson (1984) suggested that information seeking behaviour has both a strong negative correlation and positive correlation to the negative impacts and acceptance of the disease, respectively. From time to time, parents are required to understand detailed information about the disease, progress of their child, and techniques of how to take care of the patient. Sometimes such an overload of information may create a sense of helplessness and misconception. Parents will feel guilty about being incapable to provide adequate support for their child. Therefore, information seeking behaviour is essential for allaying the feelings of anxiety and uncertainty imposed by the situation. Hence, parents who are able to access more information tend to have higher levels of confidence in caring for their children.

Here are the quotes from interviewed mothers:

> 'I want someone (doctor or nurse) who can explain the treatments to me with details... Let me ask questions in a leisurely manner. Explain to me slowly. Sometimes, I don't know how to express my concerns.' [Mother A]

> 'I certainly want to have very detailed explanation about my son's condition. However, it is difficult for me to approach the nurses to ask questions. They only respond with a few statements and move to another patient. They are too busy and are not able to provide full attention to us.' [Mother B]

> 'I want to know and learn more from other parents with children currently hospitalized. Their experiences are valuable.' [Mother C]

2.2. Seeking Social Support

2.2.1. Spousal Support

There are two ways of communicating between spouses, reflected as either direct or indirect interactions. We found that spouses would discuss the progress and prognosis of their child with each other when their child has had chemotherapy. During the time of discussion, the parents might express their feelings directly by crying or being depressed. Concerning indirect interactions, spouses might not directly express their feelings to each other. Conversely, they might try to provide tangible support for each other, which included rotationally taking care of the child and taking turns doing housework. In fact, open communication between spouses is crucial for improving the marital relationship. It avoids misunderstanding as spouses may have different expectations of the treatment's outcome and prognosis.

Here is a quote of an interviewed parent:

> 'My husband's support is not explicit when my son has been hospitalized. At the beginning, he said I was not tough enough. I felt angry as I was not understood. After that, we communicated more; I realized that he didn't want me to feel sad.' [Mother E]

2.2.2. Social Support from Friends

We found that parents were reluctant to mobilize resources in their own social circles. As mentioned, parents seldom involve their friends and relatives throughout the hospitalization of their children. It can be addressed as a consequence of the parents still being influenced by the concept of fatalism and a sense of personal honour (Hull, 1992).

In eastern countries, people are deeply embedded in a concept of fatalism and a strong sense of personal honour. Fatalism is a concept that is highly advocated in Confucianism which emphasizes predetermined fate. A person who has an illness tends to accept it as fate rather than by choosing to manage the situation. Life-threatening diseases are usually regarded as a retribution or representation of sin of pre-existence. Meanwhile, a sense of personal honour is a notion that discourages weakness and fragility. The person who exposes his or her weakness in public will lose the respect of their group and the community, which is a disgraceful and embarrassing situation. A person who does something that violates the social norms would be rebuked and teased by the public (Juckett, 2005).

Here are the quotes from interviewed parents:

> 'People think it is very strange, the food has to be very clean. ... We have our difficulties... how can we explain to others? No need (to explain), very embarrassing. Actually I don't really mind. Some people may understand, but some people may gossip around.' [Mother F]

> 'I prefer to talk with those parents who have children with cancer. Other people are outsiders. They don't understand how I feel. Only those parents who have similar backgrounds can comfort me.' [Mother D]

KEY TO SUCESSFUL ADAPTATION

Therapeutic Counseling

A therapeutic counseling service is essential for helping parents to minimize their sense of guilty and unnecessary fear, to enhance their ability for coping, to facilitate their emotional expression, and to enable them to seek social support, when their child is hospitalized with cancer.

On admission, clinical nurses in the paediatric oncology ward will do a psychosocial assessment for both patients and parents. It is essential for health care professionals to assess their family structure and social support, so as to identify any high risk cases of psychosocial disturbances. Individualized nursing care plan is formulated and therapeutic counseling is given in order to minimize the negative impacts of cancer on them.

Effective counseling is composed of four elements: therapeutic environment; permission to speak; respecting the differences between the counselor and patient; and confidentiality. All parents are counseled by nurses to allay their anxiety. Those patients or parents identified as high risk are referred by clinical nurses to other counseling service. In addition, regular meetings are held in the paediatric oncology department. The doctors, nurses, clinical psychologists, social workers and pastors are present in the meeting in order to discuss the psychosocial needs of the patients and their families. In fact, nurses play an important role in counseling service and in promoting the parents' mental well-being.

Parents' Education

As mentioned, parents who can access more information related to the illness find it easier to accept the fact that their children have an illness than those who cannot access medical information. Therefore, parents' education is essential for enhancing their ability to cope with the situation. The current study showed that some parents had difficulties in communicating with health care professionals, in particular, in understanding the complex condition of patients and expressing their concerns. In addition, the high occupancy and lacking of staff in the oncology ward challenged the health care team to do their best to meet the parents' needs. Therefore, health care professionals should have a well-structured information giving strategies to satisfy the needs of those parents. Effective interventions should be developed to faciliate the process of information delivery. Training programs for nursing staff are essential to improve the standard of patient education and counseling.

In Hong Kong, clinical nurse deliver information in parents' education according to the parents' needs and ward standard protocol. Nurses should deliver the content of parent education at an appropriate dose and frequency during different stages of cancer journery. The parents' coping strategies and level of stress should be taken into consideration. Parents are encouraged to ask questions and express their concerns to nurses. Nurse provides relevant booklets, pamphlets and videos to the newly diagnosed cases. The information includes the illness progress, medication regime, treatment plan; instruction on procedure or skills performed at home, prevention of complication. Some health talks are also arranged regularly for those parents. The topics for health talks include dietary advice, late side effects of the cancer treatments, psycho-social adjustment of children, academic and family related issues. Parents are provided with access to a hotline service where a nurse specializing in paediatric oncology care is responsible for answering questions.

Parent Support Groups

In Hong Kong, some parent support groups were established for parents have children with cancer. One of the support groups is self-operated by parents, while a nurse specialist and a medical social worker serve as the coordinators. The support group holds regular meetings in the ward for parents who have children hospitalized with cancer. The group serves as a platform for parents to ventilate and express their feelings. Educational talks and clinical visits are occasionally organized by the nurse specialist. In addition, celebrations and parties are held during different festivals, such as Christmas, Chinese New Year, Easter, Mid-Autumn Festival, Mother's Day and Father's Day, etc. Such celebrations help the patients and their parents to retain a sense of social connection.

Here are the quotes from interviewed parents:

> 'When my child was admitted to the hospital, I was visited by the volunteers. It was a good experience as I felt helpless at that moment.' [Mother A]

> 'The happiest thing was to see my child playing happily in the Christmas party.' [Mother F]

Social Support

Social support can reduce or buffer the negative impacts caused by the illness (Cohen and Eillis, 1985). As mentioned, parents who have support from their immediate family members and close relatives adapt better in the problem solving stage than those who do not. However, a restricted visitor policy has been adopted in many hospitals (in both eastern and western countries) in order to minimize the occurrence of clinical infection. Hence, patients and their parents find it difficult to maintain social connections with their friends and also the community. Parents are also encouraged to mobilize their social resources, such as accepting help from relatives and friends and utilizing social services or respite care offered by non-government organizations.

Positive Thinking and Spiritual Support

Positive thinking is one of the coping strategies that enables parents to enhance their self-esteem. According to Jean Waston's philosophy of nursing, nurses are the curative factors which impact both human science and art. There are ten curative factors which include: (1) the formation of a humanistic-altruistic system of values; (2) the installation of faith-hope; (3) the cultivation of sensitivity to one's self and to others; (4) the development of a helping-trust relationship; (5) the promotion and acceptance of the expression of positive and negative feelings; (4) the systematic use of the scientific problem-solving method for decision making; (7) the promotion of interpersonal teaching-learning; (8) the provision of a supportive, protective and/or corrective mental, physical, cultural and spiritual environment; (9) assistance with the gratification of human needs; and (10) the allowance of existential-phenomenological forces(Watson, 1997).

For the instillation of faith and hope, nurses play a vital role by assisting patients and their caregivers to explore the hidden meanings of illness which are relevant to them. Therefore, as a health care professional, nurses should enable parents who have children hospitalized with cancer to explore the positive meanings of the experience. The results of our study showed that parents would usually attribute the positive meanings of illness to: (1) increasing family cohesion; (2) increasing their patience; and (3) increasing their faith in God. Illness provides parents with an opportunity to redefine their goals and values. Some parents reported that they realized the importance of having a balance in family life after their children had cancer. Concerning the increase of faith in God, some parents found that spiritual support was important for them in order to evaluate the illness in a positive manner. The parents reported that the illness of children can be viewed as a trial given by God. Therefore, nurses should allow them to address their spiritual needs whenever possible. Nurses also need to assess the resources which are available in the clinical setting and make appropriate referrals when necessary.

CONCLUSION

The study revealed that parents who have children hospitalized with cancer cope with the challenges by using different coping strategies. Parents adopted some emotional coping strategies since they are influenced by the fatalism and concept of a sense of personal honour. In addition, they also adopted a problem-solving strategy in order to control the situation. The current study indicated that parents with children hospitalized with cancer have difficulties in mobilizing the resources provided by the community and fail to seek help from their social network apart from their immediate family members. Therefore, as health care professionals, we should enhance parents' abilities to cope by implementing different interventions, which include counseling services, patient education, parent support group, encouraging them to mobilize social support, using the positive thinking skill, and providing spiritual support.

REFERENCES

Barker, G. (2007). Adolescents, social support and help-seeking behavior : An international literature review and programme consultation with recommendations for action. WHO.

Cohen S. and Willis T. A. (1985). Stress, social support, and the buffering hypothesis. *Psychology Bulletin* 98:310-57.

Felton B. J. and Revenson T. A. (1984). Coping with chronic illness: a study of illness controlability and influence of coping strategies on psychological adjustment. *Journal of Consult Clinical Psychology* 53:345-53.

Hull, M.M. (1992). Coping strategies of family caregivers in hospice homecare. *Oncology Nursing Forum*, 19(8), 1179-1187.

Juckett, G.(2005). Cross Cultural Medicine. *Amercian Family Physician,72* (11),2267-2274.

Karak, A. and Nachman, G. S. (1991). Family research on childhood chronic illness: Paediatric oncology as an example. *Journal Family Psychology*, 4:462 - 483.

Lambert, V.A. and Lambert C.E. (2008). Nurses' workplace stressors and coping strategies. *Indian Journal of Palliative Care, 14*(1), 38-44.

Lazarus, R.S., and Folkman, S. (1984). Stress, appraisal, and coping. New York: Springer.

Rowland J. H. (1990). Intrapersonal resource: coping. *Handbook of psychooncology: psychological care of the patient with cancer.* New York: Oxford University Press.

Sheridan C. L. and Radmacher S. A. (1992). Stress and health. In *Health Psychology – challenging the biomedical model.* Wiley, New York. p147-169.

Taylor S. E. (1995) Moderator of the stress experiences. *Health Psychology.* New York: McGraw-Hill.

Watson, J. (1997). The theory of human caring: Retrospective and prospective. Nursing Science Quarterly, 10(1), 49-52.

In: Pediatric Cancer
Editor: William Li

ISBN: 978-1-61942-112-7

Chapter 8

CONTINUOUS RENAL REPLACEMENT THERAPY IN CHILDREN POST-HEMATOPOIETIC STEM CELL TRANSPLANTATION

Lama Elbahlawan and R. Ray Morrison
Division of Critical Care Medicine,
St. Jude Children's Research Hospital, Memphis, Tennessee, US

ABSTRACT

Allogeneic hematopoietic stem cell transplantation (HSCT) is being utilized increasingly as a curative therapy for an array of disorders like hematologic malignancies, immunodeficiency, and inborn errors of metabolism. However, many complications that occur after transplant can have a significant negative impact on outcome and thus limit the benefit of this therapy. Acute renal failure (ARF) occurs commonly after HSCT and is associated with high risk of morbidity and mortality. Common factors associated with ARF early after HSCT include acute tubular necrosis, veno-occlusive disease, and septic shock. Conditioning regimens and total body irradiation as well as the use of nephrotoxic medications contribute to the occurrence of ARF 60 days following HSCT. Recently, continuous renal replacement therapy (CRRT) has emerged as the favored modality of renal replacement therapy in the care of critically ill children who are hemodynamically unstable. CRRT is increasingly used in the care of critically ill post-HSCT children to treat renal failure or to prevent fluid overload (FO) as FO seems to be associated with worse outcome in these patients. Studies have shown that the risk of mortality is higher when CRRT is initiated at FO>20% in critically ill children as well as post-HSCT children. In our experience, CRRT results in improved oxygenation in post-HSCT children with acute lung injury. Mean airway pressure at the end of CRRT seems to be an important prognostic factor for pediatric stem cell recipients who are mechanically ventilated because survivors have lower mean airway pressures at the end of CRRT compared to non-survivors. This high mean airway pressure at the end of CRRT is likely related to the intrinsic pulmonary process that lead to pulmonary failure rather than pulmonary edema secondary to FO. Although CRRT is associated with improved short-term outcome, long-term survival (>6 months following intensive care unit discharge) is very poor. Factors associated with lower long-term survival include higher C-reactive protein (CRP) and lower absolute neutrophil count (ANC). Prospective multi-institutional studies are needed to definitively establish prognostic factors associated with better survival. In addition, the best modality of CRRT for attenuating the inflammatory process should be investigated in this population. Protocols that delineate the appropriate time to initiate CRRT before 20% FO may also be valuable in improving outcome in this high-risk population.

INTRODUCTION

Hematopoietic stem cell transplant (HSCT) is increasingly used to treat a variety of disorders including malignancy, immunodeficiency, and inborn errors of metabolism. However, this therapy is still associated with high risk of complications and morbidities. Acute kidney injury (AKI) is common following HSCT and adversely affects short and long term outcomes of these patients [1-3]. Management of AKI when it occurs entails treating the cause leading to AKI, but supportive measures like dialysis may become essential for managing electrolyte disturbances and/or fluid overload or even uremia. Critically ill post-HSCT children with renal dysfunction or fluid overload pose a greater challenge if dialysis is needed because of frequently concomitant hemodynamic instability. Continuous renal replacement therapy (CRRT) offers the advantage of removing fluid at a slow rate that can be better tolerated in hemodynamically unstable children. This chapter will give an overview of the use of CRRT, its indications, and potential benefits in critically ill post-HSCT children. It will also discuss outcomes and highlight predictors of survival in this high-risk population when this therapy is used.

Overview of Acute Kidney Injury Post-HSCT

The incidence of AKI in patients receiving HSCT ranges from 14% in some series to as high as 73% in others [1-4]. Common factors associated with ARF early after HSCT include acute tubular necrosis, veno-occlusive disease, and septic shock. Conditioning regimens and total body irradiation as well as the use of nephrotoxic medications contribute to the occurrence of ARF within the first 60 days following HSCT. The management of AKI includes withdrawal of nephrotoxic medications when possible, and prevention of hypotension and hypoxia to avoid perpetuating kidney injury. Diuretics like furosemide are often used intermittently or as a continuous drip to manage fluid overload and enhance diuresis. However, in post-HSCT children, prevention of fluid overload is particularly challenging. On one hand, most of these patients manifest some degree of systemic inflammatory response syndrome (SIRS) following transplant that is triggered by the conditioning regimen of total body irradiation and chemotherapy. On the other hand, these patients often receive high amounts of fluid as part of their therapy and nutrition, and even adequate urine output of more than 2ml/kg/hr may be insufficient to prevent fluid overload. When diuretic therapy and fluid restriction fail, CRRT is usually considered in the intensive care unit (ICU) to prevent further fluid overload. The most common reasons for initiating CRRT in children with stem cell transplant are fluid overload with electrolyte imbalance (49%), followed by fluid overload alone (39%), and then electrolyte imbalance (8%) [5]. Therefore, in some instances, CRRT is initiated even before the occurrence of ARF, strictly in order to manage fluid overload when diuretic therapy fails.

Modalities of CRRT

Modern CRRT usually involves draining blood from the venous circulation, followed by pumping the blood through a circuit with a semipermeable membrane (or filter), and then returning it to the venous circulation, usually via a large caliber double lumen central catheter. There are different modalities of CRRT based on the mechanism of solute removal. Most commonly used modalities are continuous venovenous hemofiltration (CVVH), continuous venvenous hemodialysis (CVVHD), continuous venovenous hemodiafiltration (CVVHDF). CVVH clears solute by convection, CVVHD by diffusion, and CVVHDF by both convection and diffusion.

In CVVH, fluid moves across a semipermeable membrane down a hydrostatic pressure gradient. During convective treatment, high-flux membranes used that are highly permeable to water as well as low and middle molecular weight solutes (in the range of 1000-12,000 Daltons). Solute clearance during CVVH is determined by the blood flow through the circuit, the hydrostatic pressure across the semipermeable membrane, and the filtration fraction (the ratio of ultrafiltrate production to filter blood flow, which is also affected by plasma oncotic pressure and hematocrit). The ultrafiltrate generated on the effluent side of the membrane is replaced with replacement fluid that can be administered pre- filter (pre-dilution) or post-filter (post-dilution).

In CVVHD, a dialysis solution is pumped in the opposite direction to patient blood flow (counter-current), resulting in diffusion of electrolytes across the membrane down a concentration gradient.

CVVHDF modality uses the 2 techniques of CVVH and CVVHD.

The most commonly used modality in post-HSCT children as reported by the prospective pediatric CRRT registry group is CVVHD (43%), followed by CVVH (37%), and then CVVHDF (20%) [5].

Anticoagulation

Anticoagulation during CRRT is important to prevent clotting of the CRRT circuit. The two most common used methods for anticoagulation are either unfractionated heparin or citrate. In patients at higher risk of bleeding, citrate is superior to heparin because it doesn't result in systemic anticoagulation, but rather anticoagulant effect is limited solely to the circuit. Both heparin and citrate offer effective anticoagulation. The prospective pediatric CRRT registry reported similar circuit lives with heparin and citrate (mean 42.1 versus 44.7 h respectively), both of which were superior to no anticoagulation (mean 27 h, $P<0.005$) [6]. However, patients receiving heparin had an increased risk of significant bleeding whereas patients receiving citrate did not. Therefore, in post-HSCT children who are at higher risk of bleeding for multiple reasons like thrombocytopenia and liver dysfunction, we recommend the use of citrate rather than heparin for anticoagulation. A continuous drip of citrate is infused at the time of initiation of the CRRT circuit and results in anticoagulation by chelating ionized calcium. Since citrate is a small molecule, the majority of the calcium-citrate complex is freely filtered. Thus, a systemic calcium infusion is necessary to replace the calcium lost with the citrate. When using citrate, patient's ionized calcium as well as post-filter ionized calcium has to be monitored closely and titrated to keep patient's ionized calcium within a normal range and post-filer ionized calcium level of 0.25-0.5 mmol/l to prevent clotting of the circuit. Side effects of citrate include citrate lock phenomena where excess citrate binds to free calcium resulting in increased serum total calcium level and a decrease in ionized calcium. Other side effects like metabolic alkalosis or metabolic acidosis (seen in patients with liver failure who may insufficiently metabolize citrate) can occur. Since citrate is metabolized in the liver, it should be avoided or used cautiously in patients with liver failure.

Complications of CRRT

CRRT is an invasive therapy that can potentially lead to multiple complications. Hemodynamic instability can be challenging with CRRT especially since this treatment is often initiated in children in an ICU setting who may have an element of hemodynamic instability. Hypotension can occur after initiation of CRRT and may necessitate initiation of a vasoactive medication or escalation of an existing vasoactive infusion. The bradykinin-release syndrome that results in severe hypotension is now encountered far less frequently after introduction of polysulfone filters that replaced the polyacrylonitrite filters that were notorious for this syndrome. In a series of 174 critically ill children treated with CRRT, hypotension occurred in 30% of the patients [7].

Another complication that may arise is related to the venous catheterization. Santiago et al. reported 7.4% rate of complications related to catheterization for CRRT, which included most commonly hematoma at the puncture site (3.4%), hemorrhage (2.2%), and altered venous drainage of the lower limbs (3.4%) [7]. Hemorrhage can also occur particularly when heparin is used for anticoagulation of the CRRT circuit. Moreover, close monitoring of serum electrolytes should be done while using this therapy because electrolyte disturbances are common during CRRT. Hypothermia may occur secondary to extracorporeal radiant heat exchange which may necessitate the use of a warming blanket. Thermal loss during CRRT may mask fever and delay recognition of infection, so other parameters of infection should be monitored closely.

CRRT in Pediatric Stem Cell Transplant

One of the earlier studies that specifically evaluated CRRT in pediatric stem cell recipients was reported by Goldstein et al. in 2004 [8]. In this retrospective review, 26 post-HSCT children with acute renal failure and fluid overload were included. Most common etiologies for ARF were nephrotoxicity in 62% of patients, followed by septic shock with or without nephrotoxicity in 35%. Children requiring CRRT had a survival rate of 18%. The need for mechanical ventilation was associated with lower survival, in contrast, <10% FO was associated with better survival.

Another larger cohort of 51 pediatric stem cell recipients receiving CRRT was reported by the prospective pediatric CRRT registry group in 2008 [5]. The most common causes for ARF and the need for CRRT were: no single identifiable cause in 33%, respiratory insufficiency in 18%, sepsis in 16%, multi-organ dysfunction syndrome in 12%, veno-occlusive disease in 8%, hepatorenal syndrome in 8%, and drug toxicity in 8%. The most frequent vascular access for CRRT was a femoral vein catheter (88%) and internal jugular vein (10%). Fifty four % of the cohort was receiving diuretics upon initiation of CRRT. Mean % FO was 12.41 ± 3.7%. Median duration of CRRT was 10.71 ± 1.56 days. Twenty three of 51 (45%) patients survived to discharge from the ICU, however, patients with ventilatory support had a significant lower survival rate compared to non-ventilated patients (35% versus 71% respectively, P=0.05).

CRRT and Acute Lung Injury

Mechanically ventilated pediatric HSCT patients have a higher risk of mortality (as high as 76.5%) that may be related to conditioning with irradiation, prior chemotherapy, and inherent immune dysregulation after transplant [9,10]. DiCarlo et al. reported improved survival in children with cancer or bone marrow transplant when CVVH was used; however, the study was limited by the small number of patients included [11]. A retrospective study in our pediatric oncology center showed that CRRT can improve oxygenation in mechanically ventilated pediatric allogeneic HSCT patients with ALI [12]. Thirty post-HSCT pediatric patients with ALI who underwent CRRT from 1994-2006 were included in this review. CRRT was associated with significant improvement of oxygenation 24 hours and 48 hours post initiation of this therapy.

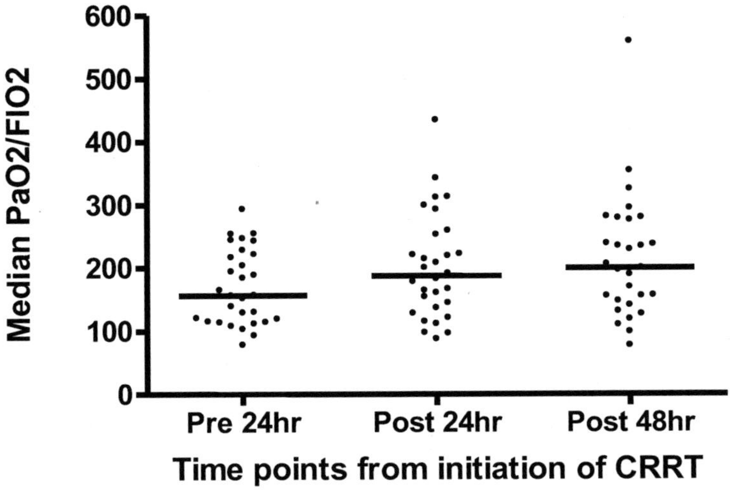

Figure 1. Median PaO_2/FiO_2 change following initiation of CRRT.

PaO_2/FiO_2 increased significantly with median increase of 31 and 43 in the 24 and 48 hrs intervals after initiation of CRRT compared to the 24 hour interval before CRRT (P=0.0008 and 0.0062 respectively). This improvement in PaO_2/FiO_2 was associated with the reduction of fluid balance after initiation of CRRT (P=0.0001).

Mean airway pressure (Paw) at the end of CRRT may relate to survival in intubated post-HSCT children. When comparing survivors to non-survivors in a pediatric HSCT cohort, Paw at initiation of CRRT was not different, however, higher mean Paw at the end of CRRT was associated with lower survival. In survivors, mean Paw at the end of CRRT was 8.7 ± 2.94 compared to 25.76 ± 2.03 ($P<0.001$) in non-survivors [5]. In our cohort of 30 post-HSCT children on CRRT, median Paw was 13 in survivors versus 17.42 in non-survivors (P=0.09) at 48 hours post initiation of CRRT and the difference may have reached statistical significance if a longer time period after CRRT was evaluated [12].

The higher Paw at the end of CRRT in non-survivors may indicate the presence of irreversible pulmonary process and not pulmonary edema as the reason for respiratory failure and non-compliant lungs. Paw may become a valuable predictor of outcome to follow once these children are started on CRRT, and failure to reduce Paw after days on CRRT may indicate a worse prognosis.

CRRT and Sepsis

CRRT use as an immunomodulator therapy in sepsis is still controversial. Convective CRRT can remove medium sized molecules from the blood (like cytokines). Although a number of studies of CVVHF in animal models of sepsis have shown reduction of cytokine and clinical improvement by using this therapy, results were not replicated in human studies [13,14]. The reduction of cytokine levels after initiation of CRRT is usually not sustainable and short lived, probably secondary to initial adsorption of cytokines onto the membrane which then become saturated. High volume hemofiltration at rates >35 ml/kg/min is more efficient in cytokine removal and appears to improve outcome in adult patients with refractory septic shock [15]. Nonetheless, this technique is associated with major practical difficulties as well as safety concerns.

On the other hand, there is concern that the early application of CRRT in sepsis-induced multiple organ failure can be harmful. In a prospective randomized trial in 12 French intensive care units, 76 patients with sepsis-induced multi-organ failure were randomized to either continuous hemofiltration (25ml/kg/hr) for a 96-hour period or to conventional management [14]. The number and severity of organ failures was significantly higher in patients undergoing continuous hemofiltration ($P<0.05$). In the above study, hemofiltration didn't impact plasma cytokine levels.

Therefore, there is not enough evidence to support the initiation of this therapy for management of sepsis as the only indication.

Controversies

Time of Initiation of CRRT

Fluid overload (FO) in ICU is associated with mortality in children receiving CRRT. Fluid overload is usually defined as the cumulative percent fluid balance (based on ICU admission weight) from ICU admission to CRRT initiation or by cumulative percent fluid balance in the 7 days prior to ICU admission. FO is calculated by the following formula: %FO= (Fluid in-Fluid out)/ (ICU admission weight)*100%. Goldstein et al. reported that in 116 children with multiple organ system dysfunction who received CRRT, the degree of fluid overload was significantly greater in non-survivors compared to survivors [16]. Children with < 20% FO had a survival of 58%, compared to 40% with FO≥ 20% ($P<0.002$). These results were comparable to another study of a large prospective series of 297 critically ill children receiving CRRT reported by the Prospective Pediatric CRRT Registry [17]. In that series, fluid overload was an independent risk factor for mortality. Children with fluid overload ≥20% had an adjusted mortality rate of 8.5 (95% CI, 2.8-25.7) compared to those with <20%. There was a 3% increase in mortality for each 1% increase in FO at CRRT initiation. Therefore, FO particularly >20% may be a valid indication to initiate CRRT if diuretic therapy and fluid restriction fails, even before overt ARF occurs.

Best Modality

Despite extensive research, the ideal method of delivering CRRT is unknown with wide variation in practice between different centers [18]. In a multicenter study of 116 children with multiple organ dysfunction syndrome (MODS), there was no significant difference in rate of survival among different modalities of CRRT [16]. In the prospective pediatric CRRT registry group report on post-HSCT children, survival rate was higher when treated with convective CRRT versus CVVHD (59% versus 27%, P<0.05) [5]. The authors speculated that the beneficial effect on survival may be attributed to better clearance of middle molecules like cytokines. However, since cytokine removal by these modalities is usually transient and non-sustainable, these results have to be interpreted with caution. The authors also speculated that this difference may be related to differences in CRRT preferences in institutions with more experienced stem cell transplant programs. Therefore, a strong recommendation of one modality versus the other can't be made based on the current research and it should be based on what the institution is most experienced in. Large prospective trials may be better-suited to answer this issue definitively.

Dose of CRRT

The optimal dose of CRRT to be used is still controversial. An earlier trial by Ronco et al. in adult patients with ARF showed improved survival with post-dilution CVVH at a rate of 35 ml/kg/hr compared to 20 mg/kg/hr [19]. However, subsequent trials failed to show the same positive effect of higher intensity CRRT. The multicenter prospective RENAL trial randomized 1508 critically ill adult patients to post-dilution CVVHDF with an effluent flow rate of either 40 ml/kg/hr or 25 ml/kg/hr [20]. Mortality rates were not statistically different between groups, indicating no survival benefit from more-intensive CRRT. Therefore, there is no convincing evidence to support the use of higher effluent flow rates since it doesn't improve survival.

Drug Clearance

Drug clearance by CRRT doesn't parallel that achieved by intermittent hemodialysis. The slow and continuous dialysate and ultrafiltrate flow rates used in CRRT can yield drug clearance similar to an analogous glomerular filtration of the native kidneys. However, developing an appropriate drug dosing regimen for patients on CRRT is not as easy as it seems. Drug clearance is influenced by many factors like the patient's renal function, dialysate/ultrafiltrate flow rates, and type of filter used. Pediatric stem cell transplant recipients frequently require antimicrobial therapy to prevent or control infection. While the pharmacokinetics of some antimicrobials like vancomycin and aminoglycosides are well characterized in patients on CRRT, other newer antimicrobials are less well studied. For example, in contrast to its clearance by intermittent hemodialysis, vancomycin has a high removal rate on CRRT due to the higher flux of volume. Therefore, close monitoring of serum drug level is important to ensure therapeutic targets are acheived.

Outcome

Mortality in children receiving CRRT is still relatively high. In a pediatric cohort of 174 children receiving CRRT, mortality rate was 35.6% [21]. Hemodynamic disturbances and the presence of multi-organ failure at the time of initiation of CRRT were associated with a higher mortality rate. Another cohort of 76 children on CRRT had an overall survival of 55.3% [22]. The presence of sepsis, MODS, and FO greater than 20% were significantly associated with higher mortality.

Short term survival of post-HSCT children undergoing CRRT ranges from 17% to 45% [5,12}. Ventilatory support confers a higher risk for mortality in this population. Interestingly higher Paw (as discussed in a previous part of this chapter) at the end of CRRT is also associated with lower survival rate.

There is paucity of reports describing the long term outcome of this therapy in this high-risk population. In fact, only one study to date by Rajasekaran et al. evaluated long term outcome after ICU discharge [23]. The cohort included 29 children who had 33 courses of CRRT. In 11/13 (33%) courses, patients survived to ICU discharge. The median duration of survival after CRRT initiation was 31 days (range, 2-405 days). Three out of the 11 patients who survived recovered adequate renal function, and 7 patients were dependent on intermittent hemodialysis. Higher serum bilirubin and blood urea nitrogen (BUN) at the time of initiation of CRRT were associated with an increased risk of death, which underscores the complexities incurred with co-morbidities other than renal failure. Improvement in PaO_2/FiO_2 at 48 hours after initiation of CRRT was significantly associated with higher survival rates. There was a 20% decrease in risk of death for every 50 point increase in the 48-hr PaO_2/FiO_2 (HR, 0.798; 95% CI, 0.656, 0.971). C reactive protein (CRP) and absolute neutrophil count (ANC) at the end of CRRT were associated with survival.

The risk of death was increased by 6% for every 1-point increase in CRP level at the end of CRRT (HR, 1.057; 95%CI, 1.023, 1.092). In addition, patients with neutropenia (as defined by ANC<500 cells/µl) at the end of CRRT had a 3 fold increase in the risk of death when compared to those without neutropenia. The primary cause of death was infection-related complication in 45% of all patients, veno-occlusive disease in 14%, and recurrence or progression of malignant disease in 10%. Only one patient survived > 6 months after initiation of CRRT.

Although outcomes of children post-HSCT requiring CRRT therapy remains relatively poor, this can be seen as an opportunity to improve this important adjunctive therapy in a very high-risk population. In the past, the survival of intubated post-HSCT patients was also dismal and now it is close to 50%. Nevertheless, CRRT is often used in the context of multi-organ dysfunction in this population, and the high risk of mortality reflects the complexity and severity of underlying illness.

FUTURE DIRECTIONS

Future studies should focus on improving outcomes when this therapy is used. Different modalities of CRRT require prospective, randomized comparison to determine which is associated with better survival, particularly since the pediatric prospective CRRT registry group on pediatric stem cell patients indicated that patients on CVVH or CVVHDF had better survival compared to patients on CVVHD. In addition, better understanding and evaluation of the pharmacokinetics of various medications while on CRRT will be helpful in guiding dosing regimens. Finally, we believe that developing protocols aimed at delineating the appropriate time to initiate CRRT (before 20% FO) would be valuable in improving outcomes in this high-risk population.

Conclusion

Pediatric CRRT is an increasingly used support technique that is both an invasive and resource intensive therapy with inherent uncertainties. Post-HSCT critically ill children may need CRRT for multiple reasons, such as FO and electrolyte disturbance. FO affects outcome negatively and >20% FO is associated with higher risk of mortality. In addition, multi-organ dysfunction at the time of initiation of CRRT is associated with lower survival. CRRT is associated with improved short-term outcomes of mechanically ventilated post-HSCT children especially if it leads to reduction of Paw. However, long term outcome is still poor. Post-HSCT children with higher CRP or lower ANC at the end of their CRRT course have worse long term outcomes. The ongoing prospective multi-center trial by the prospective pediatric CRRT registry group continues to offer important insight into this treatment in children. It should be kept in mind that what applies to the general pediatric population may not apply to the specific post-HSCT pediatric population as HSCT patients have different disease processes that may make ARF more complicated. In addition, careful and thorough discussions with the families about prognosis and outcome have to be conducted early before this therapy is initiated. A question families frequently ask of nephrologists and intensivists alike is whether the kidneys will recover after CRRT is required. Unfortunately, there are no specific diagnostic laboratory tests that can answer this question. Non-oliguric renal failure is usually associated with better chance of renal function recovery. In our cohort of post-HSCT children on CRRT, 10% recovered adequate renal function, while 24% required intermittent hemodialysis [23]. Prevention of ARF should remain a main focus in pediatric stem recipients with less toxic preparative chemotherapy regimens, monitoring drug levels of nephrotoxic medications, and prompt treatment of hypotension and hypoxia. When FO occurs, consideration of CRRT should not be delayed as its earlier initiation may result in improved outcomes in this high-risk population.

References

[1] Parikh CR, McSweeney PA, Korular D, Ecder T, Merouani A, Taylor J, Slat-Vasquez V, Shpall EJ, Jones RB, Bearman SI, Schrier RW. Renal

dysfunction in allogeneic hematopoietic cell transplantation. *Kidney Int* 2002;62: 566-573.

[2] Parikh CR, Schrier RW, Storer B, Diaconescu R, Sorror ML, Maris MB, Maloney DG, McSweeney P, Storb R, Sandmaier BM. Comparison of ARF after myeloablative and nonmyeloablative hematopoietic cell transplantation. *Am. J. Kidney Dis*. 2005; 45: 502-509.

[3] Hingorani SR, Guthrie K, Batchelder A, Schoch G, Aboulhosn N, Manchion J, McDonald GB. Acute renal failure after myeloablative hematopoietic cell transplant: incidence and risk factors. *Kidney Int* 2005; 67:272-277.

[4] Hosing C, Nash R, McSweeney P, Mineishi S, Seibold J, Griffith LM, Shulman H, Goldmuntz E, Mayes M, Parikh CR, Crofford L, Keyes-Elstein L, Furst D, Steen V, Sullivan KM. Acute kidney injury in patients with systemic sclerosis participating in hematopoietic cell transplantation trials in the United States. *Biol. Blood Marrow Transplant* 2011; 17:674-681.

[5] Flores FX, Brophy PD, Symons JM, Fortenberry JD, Chua AN, Alexander SR, Mahan JD, Bunchman TE, Blowey D, Somers MJ, Baum M, Hackbarth R, Chand D, McBryde K, Benfield M, Goldstein SL. Continuous renal replacement therapy (CRRT) after stem cell transplantation. A report from the prospective pediatric CRRT Registry *Group. Pediatr. Nephrol* 2008; 23: 625-630.

[6] Brophy PD, Somers MJ, Baum MA, Symons JM, McAfee N, Fortenberry JD, Rogers K, Barnett J, Blowey D, Baker C, Bunchman TE, Goldstein SL. Multi-centre evaluation of anticoagulation in patients receiving continuous renal replacement therapy (CRRT). *Nephrol. Dial Transplant* 2005; 20: 1416-1421.

[7] Santiago MJ, López-Herce J, Urbano J, Solana MJ, del Castillo J, Ballestero Y, Botrán M, Bellón JM. Complications of continuous renal replacement therapy in critically ill children: a prospective observational evaluation study. *Crit. Care* 2009; 13 (6):R184.

[8] Michael M, Kuehnle I, Goldstein SL. Fluid overload and acute renal failure in pediatric stem cell transplant patients. *Pediatr. Nephrol* 2004; 19: 91-95.

[9] Lamas A, Otheo E, Ros P, Vázquez JL, Maldonado MS, Muñoz A, Martos I. Prognosis of child recipients of hematopoietic stem cell transplantation requiring intensive care. *Intensive Care Med.* 2003; 29:91-96.

[10] Tamburro RF, Barfield RC, Shaffer ML, Rajasekaran S, Woodard P, Morrison RR, Howard SC, Fiser RT, Schmidt JE, Sillos EM. Changes in outcomes (1996-2004) for pediatric oncology and hematopoietic stem cell transplant patients requiring invasive mechanical ventilation. *Pediatr. Crit. Care Med.* 2008; 9: 270-277.

[11] DiCarlo JV, Alexander SR, Agarwal R, Schiffman JD. Continuous veno-venous hemofiltration may improve survival from acute respiratory distress syndrome after bone marrow transplantation or chemotherapy. *J. Pediatr. Hematol. Oncol.* 2003; 25: 801-805.

[12] Elbahlawan L, West NK, Avent Y, Cheng C, Liu W, Barfield RC, Jones DP, Rajasekaran S, Morrison RR. Impact of continuous renal replacement therapy on oxygenation in children with acute lung injury after allogeneic hematopoietic stem cell transplantation. *Pediatr. Blood Cancer* 2010; 55: 540-555.

[13] Cole L, Bellomo R, Hart G, Journois D, Davenport P, Tipping P, Ronco C. A phase II randomized, controlled trial of continuous hemofiltration in sepsis. *Crit. Care Med.* 2002; 30: 100-106.

[14] Payen D, Mateo J, Cavaillon JM, Fraisse F, Floriot C, Vicaut E; Hemofiltration and Sepsis Group of the Collège National de Réanimation et de Médecine d'Urgence des Hôpitaux extra-Universitaires. Impact of continuous venovenous hemofiltration on organ failure during the early phase of severe sepsis: a randomized controlled trial. *Crit. Care Med.* 2009; 37: 803-810.

[15] Honore PM, Jamez J, Wauthier M, Lee PA, Dugernier T, Pirenne B, Hanique G, Matson JR. Prospective evaluation of short-term, high-volume isovolemic hemofiltration on the hemodynamic course and outcome in patients with intractable circulatory failure resulting from septic shock. *Crit. Care Med.* 2000; 28: 3581-3587.

[16] Goldstein SL, Somers MJ, Baum MA, Symons JM, Brophy PD, Blowey D, Bunchman TE, Baker C, Mottes T, McAfee N, Barnett J, Morrison G, Rogers K, Fortenberry JD. Pediatric patients with multi-organ dysfunction syndrome receiving continuous renal replacement therapy. *Kidney Int* 2005; 67: 653-8.

[17] Sutherland SM, Zappitelli M, Alexander SR, Chua AN, Brophy PD, Bunchman TE, Hackbarth R, Somers MJ, Baum M, Symons JM, Flores FX, Benfield M, Askenazi D, Chand D, Fortenberry JD, Mahan JD, McBryde K, Blowey D, Goldstein SL. Fluid overload and mortality in children receiving continuous renal replacement therapy: the prospective

pediatric continuous renal replacement therapy registry. *Am. J. Kidney Dis.* 2010; 55: 316-325.

[18] Symons JM, Chua AN, Somers MJ, Baum MA, Bunchman TE, Benfield MR, Brophy PD, Blowey D, Fortenberry JD, Chand D, Flores FX, Hackbarth R, Alexander SR, Mahan J, McBryde KD, Goldstein SL. Demographic characteristics of pediatric continuous renal replacement therapy: a report of the prospective pediatric continuous renal replacement therapy registry. *Clin. J. Am. Soc. Nephrol.* 2007; 2: 732-738.

[19] Ronco C, Bellomo R, Homel P, Brendolan A, Dan M, Piccinni P, La Greca G. Effects of different doses in continuous veno-venous haemofiltration on outcomes of acute renal failure: a prospective randomised trial. *Lancet* 2000 1; 356: 26-30.

[20] RENAL Replacement Therapy Study Investigators, Bellomo R, Cass A, Cole L, Finfer S, Gallagher M, Lo S, McArthur C, McGuinness S, Myburgh J, Norton R, Scheinkestel C, Su S. Intensity of continuous renal-replacement therapy in critically ill patients. *N. Engl. J. Med.* 2009 22; 361: 1627-1638.

[21] Santiago MJ, López-Herce J, Urbano J, Solana MJ, del Castillo J, Ballestero Y, Botrán M, Bellón JM. Clinical course and mortality risk factors in critically ill children requiring continuous renal replacement therapy. *Intensive Care Med.* 2010; 36: 843-849.

[22] Hayes LW, Oster RA, Tofil NM, Tolwani AJ. Outcomes of critically ill children requiring continuous renal replacement therapy. *J. Crit Care* 2009; 24: 394-400.

[23] Rajasekaran S, Jones DP, Avent Y, Shaffer ML, Elbahlawan L, Henderson N, Barfield RC, Morrison RR, Tamburro RF. Outcomes of hematopoietic stem cell transplant patients who received continuous renal replacement therapy in a pediatric oncology intensive care unit. *Pediatr. Crit. Care Med.* 2010; 11: 699-706.

INDEX

A

absolute neutrophil count (ANC), xv, 134, 143
academic performance, 18, 24, 58, 90, 100
academic progress, 24
access, 125, 127, 128, 138
accommodation, 60, 61
accountability, x, 32, 49
acute lung injury, xiv, 134, 146
acute lymphoblastic leukemia, 5, 11, 53
acute renal failure, 138, 145, 147
Acute renal failure (ARF), xiv, 133
acute respiratory distress syndrome, 146
acute tubular necrosis, xiv, 133, 135
adaptation, 25, 123
adjunctive therapy, 143
adjustment, 27, 32, 47, 51, 71, 73, 130
adolescents, 9, 11, 13, 27, 28, 29, 50, 51, 52, 53, 68, 72, 73, 82, 92, 93, 95, 107, 115, 116, 117, 118
adsorption, 140
adult cancers, vii, 1, 2, 7
adulthood, 10, 67, 68, 73, 79, 94, 99
adults, 17, 27, 32, 57, 59, 68, 71, 77, 82, 92
advancement, vii, xi, 1, 8, 49, 56, 70
advancements, 6
adverse effects, x, 55, 57, 76, 99, 113
aetiology, 9
Africa, 5
age, x, 3, 10, 12, 17, 23, 28, 32, 38, 39, 41, 42, 52, 62, 63, 65, 66, 67, 68, 70, 71, 72, 73, 81, 82, 83, 84, 85, 86, 88, 89, 102, 106, 107, 108, 117
agencies, 7
aggressiveness, 121
ALI, 138
alienation, 20, 47
aminoglycosides, 142
ANC, xv, 134, 143, 144
anger, 17, 32, 57, 68, 78
angiogenesis, 11
anisotropy, 12
ANOVA, xiii, 41, 42, 43, 98, 108, 109, 111, 112
antibody, 11
anticoagulant, 136
anticoagulation, 136, 137, 145
antimicrobial therapy, 142
anxiety, ix, x, 16, 17, 20, 31, 32, 33, 34, 35, 36, 37, 40, 41, 42, 43, 44, 45, 47, 51, 56, 57, 70, 72, 78, 88, 92, 93, 94, 99, 103, 115, 120, 124, 127
appetite, 20, 33
assessment, xiii, 22, 26, 57, 69, 82, 98, 104, 105, 107, 122, 126
assessment tools, 22
assimilation, 60, 61
astrocytoma, 6, 11
atmosphere, 38
attitudes, 102

autonomy, 49
avoidance, 18, 58, 59, 60, 68, 100, 121, 123
awareness, x, 17, 32, 49, 70, 98, 101

B

background information, 124
badminton, 106
base, 72
behaviors, 93, 116
beneficial effect, xii, 78, 97, 99, 103, 141
benefits, 35, 121
bias, 38, 84
bilirubin, 142
biopsy, viii, 2, 6
bleeding, 17, 136
blood, 35, 53, 135, 136, 140, 142
blood flow, 136
blood urea nitrogen, 142
bonds, 90
bone, 2, 6, 17, 35, 51, 56, 138, 146
bone marrow, 17, 35, 51, 56, 138, 146
bone marrow transplant, 17, 35, 51, 56, 138, 146
bone tumors, 2
bradykinin, 137
brain, 2, 6, 7, 11, 12, 17, 51, 103, 115
brain tumor, 2, 6, 7, 11, 51, 115
brainstem, 11

C

C reactive protein, 143
calcium, 137
caliber, 135
cancer cells, 11
cancer screening, xi, xii, 17, 33, 75, 97
cancer treatment, x, 17, 21, 22, 25, 34, 55, 56, 57, 71, 88, 111
carcinoma, 2, 5
caregivers, viii, 15, 18, 78, 129, 130
case studies, 36
case study, 53
categorization, 84, 85
catheter, 135, 138
Census, 100, 115
central nervous system, 7, 11
challenges, xiv, 11, 120, 122, 123, 130
chemical, 103
chemotherapeutic agent, 6
chemotherapy, ix, x, xi, 3, 6, 7, 11, 17, 22, 25, 29, 31, 33, 48, 52, 54, 55, 56, 57, 64, 75, 76, 77, 90, 99, 111, 125, 135, 138, 144, 146
Chicago, 41, 63, 84, 108
childhood cancers, vii, x, 1, 2, 3, 4, 5, 6, 7, 8, 33, 55, 76
China, 1, 9, 15, 31, 49, 52, 55, 75, 97, 115, 119
chromosome, 7
chronic illness, 66, 130
circulation, 135
clarity, 84
classification, vii, 1, 3
clinical application, 82, 107
clinical trials, 6
clone, 5
coding, 84, 85
cognitive abilities, 76
cognitive ability, 67, 68, 79
cognitive capacities, 17, 20, 21, 26, 32, 37, 57, 61, 78, 79
cognitive development, 34, 59, 60, 61, 63, 67, 69, 70, 83, 84
cognitive theory, 103, 115
colon, 3
combination therapy, 7
communication, 84, 125
communication skills, 84
community, xiii, xiv, 28, 53, 95, 98, 102, 104, 106, 114, 119, 121, 126, 129, 130
community support, xiii, 98, 114
complexity, 143
compliance, 34, 35
complications, xiv, 8, 17, 38, 133, 134, 137
computed tomography, 11
computer, ix, 31, 32, 36, 37, 38, 39, 41, 42, 44, 45, 47, 48, 49, 50
conditioning, 135, 138
confidentiality, 19, 41, 63, 108, 122, 127

configuration, 41, 81, 106
confinement, 20, 33, 47
confrontation, 59, 69, 121
Confucianism, 18, 58, 68, 126
consensus, 84, 85
consent, 19, 21, 41, 63, 83, 108, 122
Constitution, 29
construct validity, 40, 41, 62, 81, 106, 107
construction, 61
contamination, 45
content analysis, 84, 85
continuous renal replacement therapy (CRRT), xiv, 133, 145
control group, x, xiii, 32, 37, 38, 41, 42, 43, 44, 45, 46, 98, 105, 108, 109, 112
controversial, 140, 141
cooperation, 9
coping strategies, vii, xi, xiv, 54, 56, 59, 62, 63, 65, 66, 67, 68, 69, 70, 71, 73, 92, 115, 120, 121, 122, 124, 127, 129, 130
coronary heart disease, 103
correlation, 24, 25, 63, 65, 66, 84, 85, 89, 124
correlation coefficient, 63, 65, 84, 85
correlations, ix, xii, 16, 22, 76, 85, 88
cost, 8
cough, 8
cough suppressant, 8
counseling, xiv, 120, 124, 126, 127, 130
C-reactive protein (CRP), xv, 134
creative thinking, 18, 58, 100
creativity, 18, 58, 100
crises, 70
cross-sectional study, viii, x, 16, 19, 21, 56, 61, 79, 88
CRP, xv, 134, 143, 144
CSF, 11
cultivation, 129
cultural beliefs, 95
cultural differences, 58, 99
cultural values, 116
culture, 18, 58
cure, 10, 17
curriculum, 100
cyclophosphamide, 10
cytokines, 140, 141

D

data analysis, 41, 63, 71, 84, 85, 108
data collection, 37, 38, 50
deficit, 69, 72
deformation, 12
delinquency, 95
demographic characteristics, 106
demographic data, 19, 21, 41, 62, 63, 79, 81, 83, 89, 106
denial, 69, 122
dentist, xvii
depression, ix, xii, 16, 20, 22, 23, 25, 27, 28, 33, 46, 47, 51, 52, 53, 57, 72, 76, 77, 87, 88, 90, 91, 92, 93, 94, 99, 103, 117
depressive symptoms, ix, x, xii, xiii, 16, 20, 21, 22, 23, 25, 31, 32, 33, 34, 36, 40, 41, 42, 43, 45, 46, 48, 49, 76, 77, 81, 85, 87, 88, 89, 91, 94, 98, 101, 103, 104, 106, 108, 109, 110, 111, 112, 113
developed countries, vii, 1, 3, 6, 8
developing countries, 8
dialogues, 84
dialysis, 134, 136
diarrhea, 8
dietary intake, 38
diffusion, 136
disability, vii, 1, 2
diseases, 18, 48, 58, 126
disposition, 82, 107
distress, 25, 35, 83, 91, 94
distribution, vii, 1, 5
diuretic, 135, 141
doctors, 127
dosage, 104
dosing, 142, 143
drainage, 137
drawing, 48
drug toxicity, 138
drugs, 77

E

East Asia, 6
Easter, 128
economic disadvantage, 95, 117
economic status, 62, 81, 106
education, xiv, 42, 62, 64, 65, 66, 81, 84, 86, 89, 100, 102, 106, 108, 114, 120, 124, 127, 130
educational attainment, 70
educators, 85
effluent, 136, 141
electrolyte, 134, 135, 137, 144
electrolyte imbalance, 135
emotion, xi, xiv, 56, 59, 60, 62, 65, 67, 68, 69, 71, 104, 120, 121, 122
emotional distress, xi, 34, 56, 69
emotional reactions, 71
emotional responses, 26, 47, 121, 124
empirical studies, vii
empowerment, xii, 98, 101, 102, 104, 105, 108, 111, 113, 114
encouragement, 90
endocrine, xi, 7, 75, 76, 99
endurance, 90
energy, 39, 48
environment, 3, 39, 45, 50, 60, 61, 121, 127, 129
environmental factors, 4
environments, 34, 39
Epstein Barr, 4, 9
Epstein-Barr virus, 9
equipment, 50
estrangement, 33
ethics, 19, 21, 41, 63, 108
ethnic groups, vii, 1, 5
evidence, x, xiii, 5, 9, 12, 23, 32, 34, 36, 40, 46, 48, 49, 50, 53, 55, 60, 62, 68, 70, 77, 79, 81, 88, 98, 101, 103, 107, 112, 113, 114, 140, 141
evolution, 113
excision, viii, 2, 6, 7
exercise, 101, 103, 117
experimental design, 38
expertise, xvii
exposure, 5, 6, 46, 112

F

factor analysis, 40, 41, 62, 81, 106, 107
faith, 114, 129
families, viii, xiii, 2, 8, 29, 74, 93, 95, 100, 116, 119, 120, 127, 144
family functioning, 100
family life, 129
family members, viii, 15, 18, 63, 78, 128, 130
family relationships, 90
fatalism, xiv, 18, 58, 68, 120, 126, 130
fear, 17, 32, 38, 47, 48, 57, 78, 90, 92, 115, 122, 124, 126
feelings, 33, 57, 60, 78, 88, 122, 124, 125, 128, 129
fever, 17, 22, 57, 137
filters, 137
filtration, 136, 142
financial, 120
flexibility, 39
fluid, xiv, 134, 135, 136, 138, 139, 140
fluid balance, 139, 140
fluid overload (FO), xiv, 134
food, 126
football, 39, 106
force, 78
Ford, 117
formal operational stage, 63, 67, 68, 79
formation, 129
formula, 140
foundations, 115
fragility, 126
funding, 7

G

gender differences, 66, 67, 73
generalizability, 70
genes, 5
genetics, 9
glandular tissues, vii, 1, 2, 3
glioma, 6

God, 129
Greece, 28, 52
group work, 94, 117
grouping, 84
growth, xi, 11, 35, 47, 49, 56, 60, 71, 75, 76, 99, 103, 121
growth factor, 11
guidelines, 44, 109
guilty, 124, 126

H

hair, 20, 22
hair loss, 20, 22
health, x, xi, xiii, 23, 24, 25, 27, 28, 29, 31, 32, 33, 34, 36, 48, 51, 57, 69, 71, 72, 73, 75, 76, 77, 78, 82, 92, 93, 98, 99, 105, 107, 111, 114, 115, 116, 117, 118, 123, 124, 126, 127, 128, 129, 130, 131
health care, x, xii, xiii, 25, 28, 31, 32, 34, 36, 51, 69, 72, 76, 77, 78, 92, 98, 105, 111, 114, 117, 123, 124, 127, 129, 130
health care professionals, xii, xiii, 25, 34, 36, 69, 76, 77, 92, 98, 105, 111, 114, 123, 124, 127, 130
health care system, 32
health education, 105
health problems, xi, 75, 76, 99
health promotion, 105
hearing impairment, 7
heart failure, 8
helplessness, 17, 32, 57, 124
hematocrit, 136
hematoma, 137
hemodialysis, 135, 142, 144
hemorrhage, 137
hepatitis, 4, 9, 76
hepatitis a, 4
hepatocellular carcinoma, 4
hepatorenal syndrome, 138
HIV, 9
HM, 72
homogeneity, 41, 42, 108
hospice, viii, 2, 8, 130
hospitalization, viii, 16, 24, 25, 26, 29, 33, 34, 35, 39, 41, 47, 70, 96, 126
hostility, 68, 121
HSCT, xiv, 133, 134, 135, 136, 138, 139, 141, 142, 143, 144
human, 9, 50, 129, 131, 140
husband, 124, 125
hygiene, 38
hypotension, 135, 137, 144
hypothesis, 130
hypoxia, 135, 144

I

ideal, 141
identification, 84, 85, 91
identity, 105
image, viii, 1, 6, 11, 94, 117
image guided radiation therapy, viii, 1, 6
immune function, 27, 51, 72
immunity, 5
immunodeficiency, xiv, 4, 133, 134
immunomodulator, 140
incidence, 2, 5, 7, 17, 40, 81, 106, 135, 145
income, 27, 51, 92
incubation period, 4
individual differences, 70
individuals, 53, 58, 99
infection, 5, 27, 47, 49, 51, 72, 90, 128, 137, 142, 143
infectious agents, 4
infertility, 76
inflammation, 3
influenza, 50
information seeking, 124
information sharing, 63
infrastructure, 106
inhibition, 18, 58, 100
inhibitor, 7
initiation, 136, 137, 138, 139, 140, 142, 143, 144
injury, 6, 134, 135, 145
institutions, 141
intellectual disabilities, 39, 53
intelligence, 73, 94

intensity modulated radiation therapy (IMRT), viii, 1, 6
intensive care unit, xv, 134, 135, 140, 147
interaction effect, 42, 44, 112
interaction effects, 112
internal consistency, 40, 41, 62, 81, 106, 107
interpersonal communication, 102
interpersonal skills, xiii, 98, 112, 113
intervention, xi, xii, 12, 34, 36, 37, 38, 40, 42, 44, 45, 47, 50, 52, 53, 56, 58, 69, 70, 93, 97, 98, 99, 104, 108, 109, 110, 112, 114, 116
intervention strategies, 70
intonation, 84
ionized calcium level, 137
irradiation, xiv, 6, 7, 57, 77, 99, 133, 135, 138
isolation, 35
issues, viii, 10, 15, 18, 19, 20, 25, 28, 33, 34, 36, 45, 47, 48, 58, 72, 73, 78, 90, 99, 100, 117, 128

K

kidney, 134, 135, 145
kidneys, 142, 144

L

laboratory tests, 144
latency, 3
lead, vii, x, xii, xv, 1, 2, 4, 17, 33, 39, 55, 88, 97, 102, 103, 134, 137
learned helplessness, 47
learning, 7, 19, 21, 32, 37, 38, 61, 79, 89, 105, 129
learning difficulties, 89
leisure, 39, 47, 53, 102, 106
leisure time, 53
leukemia, 3, 5, 7, 11, 17, 29, 64, 85, 96
life experiences, 122
light, vii, viii, 15, 19, 48
Likert scale, 40, 81, 82, 106, 107
liver, 3, 136
liver failure, 137
locus, 60, 67, 70, 72, 94
logical reasoning, 67, 68, 79
longitudinal study, 18, 28, 58, 66, 73, 100, 118
loss of appetite, 22, 57
lumbar puncture, 35, 52
lumen, 135
lymphoid, 4
lymphoma, 3, 4, 5, 6, 9, 11, 17, 22, 64, 85

M

majority, 6, 35, 36, 103, 137
malignancy, vii, 1, 3, 5, 10, 134
management, 10, 104, 135, 140
marital conflict, 120
market share, 7
matter, 12
MB, 145
measurement, 8, 73
measurements, 105
mechanical ventilation, 138, 146
median, 139, 142
medical, viii, ix, x, xi, xvii, 2, 15, 17, 18, 19, 21, 23, 25, 26, 31, 32, 33, 34, 35, 36, 37, 38, 42, 45, 47, 50, 55, 56, 57, 59, 61, 69, 73, 75, 76, 77, 78, 79, 83, 85, 86, 99, 111, 117, 120, 127, 128
medical care, 117
medication, 127, 137
medicine, xvii
medulloblastoma, 6, 11
membranes, 136
memory, 89
memory loss, 89
mental ability, 103
mental health, 18, 28, 58, 72, 93, 100, 116, 117
mentoring, 94, 117
metabolic acidosis, 137
metabolic alkalosis, 137
metabolism, xiv, 133, 134
metabolized, 137
methodology, 6

misconceptions, vii, 1, 2, 35, 48
misunderstanding, 125
models, 140
modifications, xiii, 98, 114
mole, 106
molecular biology, 7
molecular weight, 136
molecules, 7, 11, 140, 141
monoclonal antibody, 7
mood states, 103
morbidity, viii, xiv, 2, 8, 133
morphine, 8
mortality, xiv, 12, 17, 133, 138, 140, 142, 143, 144, 146, 147
mortality rate, 17, 141, 142
mortality risk, 147
MR, 11, 147
multidimensional, 24, 29, 95, 118
multiple regression, 23, 85, 87, 89
multiple regression analysis, 23, 85, 89
mutation, vii, 1, 4

N

nasopharynx, 3
nausea, 17, 20, 22, 33, 57
negative emotions, 121
negative influences, xiii, 119, 120
nephroblastoma, 3, 6
nephrotoxic medications, xiv, 133, 135, 144
nervous system, 11
neuroblastoma, 3, 7, 11, 12
neurotransmitters, 103
neutropenia, 143
norepinephrine, 103
normal development, 34
nuclear family, 100
nurses, ix, x, xiv, 16, 25, 26, 32, 34, 48, 49, 55, 56, 57, 70, 71, 78, 91, 120, 122, 125, 126, 127, 129
nursing, ix, xi, xiv, 16, 34, 36, 41, 45, 48, 49, 51, 52, 53, 56, 69, 70, 72, 83, 120, 127, 129
nursing care, 41, 48, 49, 52, 69, 127
nutrition, 135

O

obedience, 18, 58, 68, 100
opportunities, 39, 47, 53
optimism, 7
organ, xi, 8, 75, 76, 99, 103, 138, 140, 141, 142, 143, 144, 146
organ toxicities, xi, 75, 76, 99
organism, 60
osteogenic sarcoma, 3
ototoxicity, 12
ox, 103

P

paediatric patients, 24, 35, 36
pain, 20, 22, 33, 40, 53, 56
palliative, viii, 2, 8, 13
parallel, 142
participants, ix, xii, xiii, 16, 20, 21, 22, 23, 33, 37, 38, 40, 41, 42, 45, 63, 64, 70, 76, 79, 80, 83, 85, 87, 89, 98, 102, 106, 108, 114
pathogenesis, 4, 5, 7, 8, 9
pathways, 11
patient care, x, 32, 52
permission, 127
personal life, 78
personality, 105
pharmacokinetics, 142, 143
Philadelphia, 7, 11, 53
Philippines, xvii
physical activity, 103, 116, 118
physical health, 28, 35, 93, 103
physical interaction, 39
physical well-being, vii, 1, 33, 34, 56, 57, 77, 89, 103
physicians, 63
Physiological, 35, 103
pilot study, xii, 28, 52, 98, 104
platform, 40, 128
playing, 39, 50, 128
pleasure, 34
PM, 146
policy, 50, 128

population, xv, 2, 5, 6, 8, 49, 50, 53, 82, 92, 94, 107, 115, 117, 134, 142, 143, 144
positive correlation, xii, 65, 67, 76, 85, 89, 124
positive feedback, 50, 113
positive mental health, 101
potential benefits, 134
preparation, x, xvii, 32, 34, 38, 42, 50, 52
preschool, 52
pressure gradient, 136
prevention, 9, 12, 49, 128, 135
primary caregivers, xiv, 51, 115, 119, 122
primary school, xiii, 98, 101, 104, 105
probability, 70
probability sampling, 70
problem behavior, 95, 117
problem solving, 59, 67, 68, 102, 121, 124, 128
problem-focused coping, 59, 60, 65, 67, 68, 69, 122
problem-solving, xiii, 69, 98, 105, 112, 113, 129, 130
professionals, 17, 25, 69, 88, 91, 99, 113, 127
prognosis, viii, xi, 2, 6, 8, 11, 17, 23, 75, 120, 125, 139, 144
psychoanalytic theories, 103
psychological distress, xiii, 36, 98, 100, 101, 103, 112
psychological health, 25, 34
psychological states, 103
psychological well-being, vii, viii, xiii, 15, 18, 28, 58, 73, 78, 95, 100, 103, 118, 119, 120
psychologist, 104
psychology, 116
psychometric properties, 40, 41, 62, 81, 82, 106, 107
psychosocial damage, x, xii, 17, 55, 97
psychosocial interventions, xii, 58, 78, 97, 98, 99, 100, 101, 114
psychosocial support, 91, 111
psychosocial well-being, vii, viii, xi, xii, 15, 16, 17, 19, 20, 23, 24, 25, 26, 28, 32, 33, 45, 47, 52, 57, 69, 72, 75, 76, 77, 78, 82, 84, 87, 88, 89, 90, 91, 93, 97, 98, 99, 101, 103, 104, 105, 111, 112, 113, 114
public housing, 105
pulmonary edema, xv, 134, 139

Q

questionnaire, 61

R

racial differences, 10
radiation, viii, xi, 1, 6, 7, 10, 75, 76, 90, 99, 111
Radiation, 11
radiation therapy, viii, 1, 6, 7, 10
radiation XE "radiation" treatment, xi, 75, 76
radiotherapy, ix, x, 11, 17, 22, 25, 31, 33, 55, 56, 76
real time, 39
reality, ix, 31, 32, 36, 37, 38, 39, 40, 41, 42, 44, 45, 47, 48, 49, 50, 51, 53
recall, 84
recognition, 137
recommendations, 36, 130
recovery, 48, 144
recreational, 48
recurrence, 57, 77, 79, 90, 143
Registry, 2, 3, 17, 27, 76, 93, 141, 145
regression, 84
regression analysis, 84
rehabilitation, 40, 51, 53
relatives, 123, 126, 128
relaxation, 69, 102
relevance, 84
reliability, 41, 62, 81, 106, 107
relief, viii, 2, 8
remission, 90
renal dysfunction, 8, 134
renal failure, xiv, 133, 143, 144, 145
renal replacement therapy, xiv, 133, 134, 145, 146, 147
replication, 72
requirements, 69

researchers, 7, 38, 84, 85
resilience, xiii, 98, 101, 103, 112, 114
resistance, 47, 90
resources, xiv, 24, 47, 79, 119, 121, 126, 129, 130
respiratory failure, 139
response, xiii, 3, 35, 38, 48, 58, 61, 62, 70, 79, 81, 98, 99, 135
restructuring, 67
retribution, 126
rights, 83
risk, ix, x, xii, xiv, 6, 9, 10, 12, 16, 20, 22, 23, 25, 31, 33, 46, 55, 76, 77, 87, 88, 90, 91, 99, 103, 111, 127, 133, 134, 136, 138, 141, 142, 143, 144, 145
risk factors, 6, 145
routines, 120

S

sadness, ix, 16, 20, 33, 45
safety, 140
SARS, 9
schemata, 60, 61
school, xiii, 24, 38, 64, 66, 68, 71, 73, 77, 82, 85, 88, 89, 90, 92, 95, 98, 100, 103, 104, 105, 107, 108, 113, 114, 116, 117
school adjustment, 95, 100, 117
science, 8, 129
secondary school students, 103
self-confidence, 122
self-control, xi, 17, 32, 45, 56, 57, 59, 67, 78, 121
self-efficacy, 103
self-empowerment, 39
self-esteem, x, xii, xiii, 27, 28, 39, 55, 57, 72, 76, 77, 82, 84, 85, 88, 89, 90, 91, 92, 93, 94, 98, 99, 101, 103, 104, 107, 108, 109, 110, 111, 112, 113, 115, 116, 117, 129
self-expression, 18, 35, 58, 100
self-worth, 103
semi-structured interviews, ix, 16, 20, 33
sensitivity, 129
sepsis, 138, 140, 142, 146
septic shock, xiv, 133, 135, 138, 140, 146
serotonin, 103
serum, 137, 142
services, xiv, 51, 116, 120, 130
sex, 39, 65, 66, 70, 86
shape, xi, 56, 70, 71
shock, 20
showing, 22, 24, 35, 41, 45, 46, 62, 81, 88, 106, 107, 112
siblings, 4, 77, 90, 100
side effects, xi, 17, 18, 22, 26, 37, 38, 57, 75, 76, 77, 78, 90, 128, 137
significance level, 37
signs, 25
Singapore, 49
social adjustment, 128
social circle, 126
social conformity, 18, 58, 100
social development, 105
social life, 90
social network, 130
social norms, 126
social resources, 129
social services, 129
social support, xi, xiv, 56, 59, 66, 67, 120, 121, 124, 126, 127, 130
social workers, 101, 105, 114, 127
socialization, 47
society, 115
software, 39
solid tumors, 3, 6, 11
solution, 121, 136
spirituality, 121
stability, 41, 81, 106
standard deviation, 42, 63, 84, 108, 110
standard error, 87
state, ix, x, 16, 20, 32, 33, 34, 36, 40, 41, 42, 43, 44, 45, 70, 103
states, 105
statistics, 9, 41, 63, 84, 108
stem cells, xviii
stigma, 8
stomatitis, 17, 57
strategy use, xi, 56, 67, 70
stratification, 6

stress, xiii, 17, 34, 35, 45, 47, 57, 59, 61, 62, 70, 73, 77, 94, 98, 101, 103, 112, 114, 120, 122, 127, 131
stressful events, 59, 122
stressors, 27, 51, 66, 67, 68, 71, 73, 130
structure, 41, 52, 60, 81, 92, 100, 106, 127
substance abuse, 95
suicidal ideation, 77
suicide, 77
surgical intervention, 57, 77, 99
surgical technique, 6
surveillance, 77, 103
survival, viii, ix, x, xi, xii, xv, 2, 6, 7, 9, 10, 15, 23, 31, 33, 55, 75, 76, 87, 97, 111, 134, 138, 139, 140, 141, 142, 143, 144, 146
survival rate, viii, ix, x, xi, xii, 2, 15, 23, 31, 33, 55, 75, 76, 87, 97, 111, 138, 141, 142, 143
survivors, vii, viii, xi, xii, xiv, 2, 8, 12, 23, 27, 28, 53, 67, 68, 72, 73, 75, 76, 77, 78, 79, 82, 83, 84, 85, 87, 88, 89, 90, 91, 93, 94, 95, 96, 97, 98, 99, 100, 101, 111, 113, 115, 116, 117, 118, 134, 139, 140
susceptibility, 47, 90
sympathy, 123
symptoms, ix, x, xii, xiii, 8, 16, 20, 21, 22, 23, 24, 25, 31, 32, 33, 34, 36, 40, 41, 42, 43, 45, 46, 48, 49, 57, 76, 77, 81, 85, 87, 88, 89, 91, 94, 98, 101, 103, 104, 106, 108, 109, 110, 111, 112, 113
syndrome, 135, 137, 138, 141, 146
systemic sclerosis, 145

T

Taiwan, 4, 49
target, 105
target population, 105
teachers, 12, 24, 101
techniques, 124, 136
technology, viii, 6, 15, 53, 111
temperature, 103
testing, 28, 36, 37, 72, 101
test-retest reliability, 62
therapeutic agents, 7
therapeutic goal, 39
therapeutic targets, 7, 142
therapy, viii, ix, x, xiv, 1, 6, 7, 11, 12, 31, 55, 87, 88, 94, 99, 111, 133, 134, 135, 137, 138, 140, 141, 142, 143, 144, 147
threats, 57, 77
thrombocytopenia, 136
time periods, xiii, 42, 43, 44, 46, 98, 108, 109, 110, 111, 112
tissue, vii, x, 1, 4, 55, 57, 77
topographic classification, vii, 1, 3
toxicity, 8, 12
training, xvii, 38, 84
transcription, 85
transformation, 4, 82, 107
transmission, 5
transplant, xiv, 133, 134, 135, 138, 141, 142, 145, 146, 147
transplant recipients, 142
transplantation, xiv, 133, 145, 146
trial, xiii, 6, 10, 36, 45, 52, 98, 104, 129, 140, 141, 144, 146, 147
tumor, vii, 1, 2, 3, 4, 6, 7, 10, 64
tumors, 6, 11
tumours, xviii, 11, 12, 17
type II error, 46
tyrosine, 7

U

UN, 142
underlying mechanisms, 6
unhappiness, 45
United, 18, 33, 145
United States, 18, 145
urine, 135
USA, xvii, 41, 63, 84, 108

V

vaccine, 4
validation, 52, 92, 94, 104, 115
vancomycin, 142
variables, 43, 45, 84, 85, 87, 89, 109

variations, 5, 6, 85
vein, 138
videos, 127
violence, 103
viral infection, 5
viral pathogens, 5
vision, 39
volleyball, 39, 106
vomiting, 17, 22, 57

W

Wales, xvii
Washington, 117
water, 136
weakness, 126
Western countries, xii, 17, 23, 24, 33, 46, 58, 77, 88, 97
WHO, 103, 118, 130
withdrawal, 122, 135
workplace, 130
World Health Organization, 24, 29, 118
worry, ix, 16, 20, 33, 45, 47

Y

yield, 142
young adults, 13, 95
young people, 104